Off to Be a Soldier, With a Daily Letter to My Wife

Luke Snyder

Introduction and Editing

By Susan Snyder

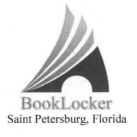

BookLocker

Saint Petersburg, Florida

Published by BookLocker.com, Inc., St. Petersburg, Florida.

Printed on acid-free paper.

BookLocker.com, Inc.
2021

First Edition

This Book is Dedicated

To Luke Snyder's Grandchildren

Amanda, Kate, Megan, Lauren, and Travis

Each of us creates history. We live out our lives in ways that reflect on others. We can reflect on our lives through stories told by family and friends, photographs, and documents. It's when we are gone that we can no longer edit that story and now it's left to others to reconstruct and interpret the experiences we may have kept private.

My Father-in-Law, Luke Snyder died in 2004. He and his wife Ruth lived in the same house for over 60 years, accumulating their history and the history of their four children. When it was time to sell the house and close this episode of their lives, it was also time to reflect on and consider what to do with the items they had collected over the years.

One of these items was a small, brown plaid, cardboard suitcase with scuffed edges and metal clasps. Found in this suitcase were approximately 330 letters, dated from July 12, 1944, to November 27th, 1945. They were all addressed to Mrs. Luke M. Snyder, Reading, Pennsylvania. They were all sent from Luke during his service in the Army during World War II; almost a letter a day for over 16 months.

To understand and appreciate the letters he wrote I feel you need to know Luke's upbringing and who he later became. He was born in 1919 in a small town founded in 1759 called Emmaus in Pennsylvania. This borough took its name from a biblical connection, a place where the disciples saw Jesus after he was crucified. Its history reflects many years of Moravian, Lutheran, and Reformed Church doctrine as well as Pennsylvania Dutch heritage; all of which influenced Luke.

Luke kept a journal during his teen years that, mundane as it might seem, documented his daily activities. He worked in his family store after school making 5-10 cents an hour and did home deliveries on his bike. He liked to play board and card games, like Parcheesi, Flinch and Rook with his Mother and Grandma. He was active in church and Sunday School plus played the clarinet in the school orchestra and band. He belonged to the Science Club and on May 17th "took a field trip to Philadelphia to visit the Hall of Natural Science, the Franklin Institute, and the Planetarium." He was also a good student, elected Class President. "Had a test in Latin. Got 100%."

Although he didn't seem to excel in sports, he took a big interest in baseball. "Listened to the All-Star game between the American League Stars and the National League Stars. The game lasted 3 hours. The American Stars won 9-7." May 28th, 1935, "The whole morning and part of the afternoon I umpired baseball games at school."

In 1936 he graduated from Ontelaunee High School, in Leesport, Pa. and went on to Ursinus College to get his Bachelor's Degree in Chemistry in 1941. From there he was hired at Carpenter Technology Corporation which made specialty steel and worked there for 43 years.

For more than 60 years he was a devoted church member of Trinity UCC in his hometown of Leesport, Pa. He took on roles of Sunday School teacher, Consistory member, and church elder.

He recognized his civic duty in politics and became a committeeman for Ontelaunee Township and later served as Vice Chairman of the Berks County Democratic Committee for several years. In 1985 he served as acting Party Chairman for a month. He also served as Township Auditor for 10 years and worked-part time as a tipstaff at the Berks County Courthouse.

Luke's umpiring career took off right after his return from the war where he began umpiring scholastic baseball games in 1946. He averaged 150 scholastic, collegiate, and sandlot baseball games a year. This passion went on for 33 years.

I'm including this accolade because it reinforces his "love of country" and his fellow man. He was a 32nd Degree Mason and more than a 50-year member of the Patriotic Order Sons of America. He was also a longtime member of the Independent Order of Odd Fellows.

Amid all the above passions and careers, his greatest passion was his family. He married his "Sweetest, Dearest, Darling" Ruth in 1939. There's some speculation that they eloped to Virginia, but neither of them would ever go into detail on the subject. They had difficulty starting a family but went on to have 3 sons and a daughter. His children, grandchildren, and in-laws will attest to his exuberance in announcing his love of family, wherever he went, and to whoever would listen.

I'm not trying to portray Luke as someone who gained great acclaim, he wasn't. Just a simple man living out his dreams and doing what he felt was expected of him. He was a small-town man; before the Army, he hardly traveled farther than New York City. He didn't want to leave home but accepted fully his duty to serve and believed he would try his best to do it well.

His words here are written exactly as he wrote them. His spelling and most times his penmanship were spot on so it made it pretty easy to interpret. His letters could run sometimes 7 pages, and I needed a magnifier to read some of the small print, especially on his V-Mail.

I did choose to shorten the letters in two ways. One was to omit many of his long and repetitive salutations, expressions of love, and closings of endearment he added to every letter. Some of these would include "Gee, but I love my Honey so very much," "I wish you knew how much you mean to me,"

"Gosh, I'm thinking of you all the time" and "I love you with my heart and soul."

The other omission is related to his daily roll call of the letters and packages, he received. He would describe how many letters, from whom, all packages, and what the contents were. I felt this was more than anybody would want to endure reading, but add it to your thoughts when reading each day because it was a significant part of almost every letter written. The only exception would be when he was short of time or too exhausted, then it might be V-Mail which limited greatly the message he could write.

The Selective Service and Training Act was a peacetime draft enacted in September 1940 and revised after the U.S. entered World War II, whereby men aged 18 to 45 were subject to military service for a term of duty that could be longer than twelve months. Since Luke was attending Ursinus College from 1936 to 1941 he was probably classified 1-D (deferred student) fit for general military service.

Army Induction then Basic Training at Camp Barkeley

[Sunday] July 9th, 1944 (written on a postcard, picturing the Reception Center-Final Inspection After Clothing Issue-Cumberland, Pa.)1

Dear Hon,

Just got back from chow! Must soon get some more tests. Visitors are allowed 7-9 PM weekdays and 9 AM to 9 PM on Sundays. Everything O.K. Don't write while I'm here. Love Luke

---

[1] Fort Indiantown Gap Reception Center processed more than 90% of Central Pa. inductees. Civilian skills and aptitude tests were given and entered onto a qualification card and sent to respective training centers.

[Wednesday] July 12th (9:30 AM)

Gosh, I sure do love you, I think you're the grandest wife in all the world.

By gosh, they keep you busy. Didn't get to bed until midnight and got up at 4:45 and we were going all day Tuesday.

I think I'll call up tonight if I get the time and if you want to you can give me an idea of when you can come up if you do at all.

How's driving coming? Did you get your learner's permit yet?

Did you hear anything yet in regards to Howard?[2]

My interview was quite good. They gave me special mention as a chemist in the organic or inorganic line, also a skilled musician and a postal clerk. After all that I guess I'll get in the ground forces. Ha! Ha!

Eats are good.

Enclosed find allotment papers and insurance copy. Keep them.

Love and Kisses Luke XXXXXXXXXX

[Thursday] July 13th

My Dearest Sweetest Hon Bun,

Gosh, but they really keep you busy. There's a rumor that a number of us will be on K.P. tomorrow.

Gee whiz, you'll never know how glad I was to see all of you last night. All of you seemed so very nice and congenial. I hope your parents didn't mind coming up.

---

[2] Howard Snyder is the brother of Luke's wife Ruth. He enlisted in 1943 as a member of the 157th Infantry which was part of the 45th Division and had been missing in action since February 8th 1944. He had landed behind enemy lines at Anzio in Italy, January 22nd.

This morning the whole outfit got our shots. They didn't hurt so much then but my arms are pretty stiff this evening. I saw one fellow pass out.

I, together with 17 other fellows, was ordered to scrub a whole barracks. That was really something but I got a kick out of it.

This morning I was told to come up to see Major Weidner. I classed in a very special group known as a chemical laboratory technician. He thinks I'll be put in the Medical Corps or some other specialized branch.

[Monday] July 17th (Pvt. Luke M. Snyder-Camp Barkeley, Texas[3] 4:50 PM)

This is it, Ruth, Camp Barkeley, Texas. I'm not sure I know my correct address yet so don't write until I say it's O.K. We left New Cumberland at 8:45 PM Friday and arrived at Abilene, Texas at 5 AM Monday. (Pardon this writing, I'm using someone else's pen, mine is dry.)

When they say Texas is hot, they're not lying. The sun bears down. This will really take some of that excess weight off. Ha! Ha!

Today we did very little thus far. After breakfast, we were put on detail to police the grounds surrounding the barracks. After that, we were told a little about what to expect in the next few months. We get 6 weeks of military basic training

---

[3] Construction began in 1940 on a temporary U.S. Army base, southwest of the town of Abilene, Texas named Camp Barkeley. It was named after David B. Barkley, winner of the Congressional Medal of Honor during World War I, but an error in spelling occurred during formation. When in full activation it became twice the size of Abilene with about 60,000 men. Divisions here were trained in infantry and armored warfare and it was also a medical replacement training center. This base was declared surplus on March 21, 1945.

and 11 more weeks of medical basic training. Boy, what a pull!

This afternoon we're just waiting to be assigned to a barracks. They haven't decided yet where to put us.

We certainly saw the scenery coming down on the train. We had a special car that the Pullman people built especially for the transfer of troops.[4] They have three births from top to bottom, 30 men in a car. During the day they can make the beds into chairs. We came west to St. Louis on the Pennsylvania R.R. There we had a slight layover. Left there at 10:30 Sat. night. We cut across Missouri, a little of Kansas, through Oklahoma, and into Texas. We came from St. Louis to Fort Worth, Texas on the Missouri, Kansas, and Texas R.R. From Fort Worth to Abilene, we came on the Texas and Pacific R.R. It was a long ride.

How's my Honey by now? Your vacation is over too! Were you in church yesterday morning? You must go every Sunday just as before. How are your parents and grandparents? Are my parents alright too? I don't know if I can get a letter written to them tonight yet. If I don't, I'll write tomorrow.

Honey, now be sure to take care of yourself while I'm not at home, and don't worry about me. Everything is fine.

I just got the correct address and I'll put it on the envelope so you can contact me there. Ha! Ha! You know how important I am. Tell my parents I wrote and am well, safe, and healthy.

---

[4] Pullman cars were dark green with Pullman Troop Sleeper printed in gold letters. They were essentially mobile barracks which reduced time spent transporting troops. They slept 29 plus the porter, had four wash stands with hot and cold running water, bunks stacked 3 high, a drinking water cooler and two enclosed toilets. They traveled with a kitchen car which prepared the meals, the men eating at their seats or bunks.

Gosh, but I love you. I certainly know now how much I love you and need you. All my love to everyone.

[Tuesday] July 18th (7:30 PM)

Gosh, but it's hot in Texas. I believe it hit 110 degrees today. I certainly haven't lost my appetite so I don't know whether I'll lose any weight or not. The sun has reddened me quite a bit.

This morning after chow, we were issued our rifles. I now feel like a soldier. I took one apart, cleaned it, and put it together again. That took us all morning. This afternoon we had a lecture for an hour on chemical warfare.[5]

They even tell you how to fold your handkerchiefs and socks. The Army has a way for everything around here. It really keeps you on your toes. It's a wonderful thing.

I want you and my parents and Sister and Grandma to be very close and congenial with one another.

P.S. You go to that doctor. We want some additions to the family. Ha! Ha!

[Wednesday] July 19th

By gosh, I think I'm pretty good to you. I've written every day so far and it keeps me busy. I've only written to you and my parents. They certainly keep you on the go.

We get up at 6 AM which isn't bad at all. We wash, make our bunks by 6:40. Then we must stand revelry and eat at 7 AM. From 8-9, we had drilling with our rifles. From 9-10, we had lectures on maps and scales. From 11-12, we had lectures on Personal Hygiene.

---

[5] Chemical warfare was not used significantly in World War II. There was some use of phosphorus grenades that caused burns and napalm that released chemicals into the air. The troops were trained to prepared for things like mustard gas.

From 2-3, we had a test on some lectures we had. I certainly never thought I'd have tests and lectures in the Army. Of course, it all adds up to make things more interesting.

From 3-5, we had lectures and drill on gas masks. We learned how to put them on, how to inspect them, and when to use them.

The fellow that has the next bunk to me is a fellow from Emmaus, my birthplace. The Army thus far hasn't made a bad boy out of me and there are plenty of men here that are fine people, so don't think I am not behaving. Ha! Ha! I certainly hope you are still behaving.

[Thursday] July 20th

Tonight, and every Thursday night we have an air raid drill at 7:45. After the air raid drill, we had to thoroughly clean our rifles and hand them in for inspection. Mine got the O.K. in flying shape. To think that Luke Snyder has learned to dismount, clean, and know all the parts of a rifle. It's amazing, isn't it?

P.S. We had Sauer Kraut and hot dogs for supper.

[Friday] July 21st

Well, today is the first day we aren't on the go all morning. We had a lecture on sex hygiene from 8-9.

Right now, it's pouring down and I love it. It feels good not to have the sun out.

Once you or my Mother get around to it you can send me some clothes hangers. There seems to be a shortage of those things around here.

How's driving coming along? Boy, that'll be nice when my wife can drive the car. Don't forget to get the car inspected by the end of the month.

Are you, Mother and Grandmother playing Rook[6] lately? I'll bet my Mother still "cheats" doesn't she?

Gosh my Dear I love you so very much. Always remember that.

[Saturday] July 22nd

So far, we haven't done a thing yet. It's been pouring and the whole place is surrounded by mud. Tomorrow sometime we'll have to change barracks. They're moving us up in alphabetical order and put in "platoons" according to that.

I've been inquiring about you living down here. Right now, I couldn't live with you and could see you on weekends only if you'd live in Abilene. After my basic things might change and I'll inquire into the matter again.

Guess what, last night for dessert we had ice cream and I got seconds on it, and it was good.

Honey, I love you and think about you so very, very much.

[Sunday] July 23rd

After chow tonight I decided to walk to the Service Men's Club. When I walked in, I saw some stationery so I thought I'd write a letter from here. Do you mind? This is a rather nice place. They have lots of desks and "soft" chairs to sit on. They certainly try to make you feel at home. I just heard that there are about 60,000 men in Camp Barkeley including about 5,000 to 8,000 prisoners of war.[7]

---

[6] The game of Rook, produced by Parker Brothers in 1906, used a specialized deck of cards. This seemed to take it away from the standard deck of cards that might be considered gambling, although the goal of the game was bidding and trick-taking.

[7] Prisoners in the U.S. helped alleviate the overcrowding situation of prisoners in Great Britain. Under the Geneva Convention the United States was required to provide living quarters comparable to our military

Today was quite an eventful day for me. I got my first letter from home. Mother had sent it Friday at noon and I got it at noon today. It was sent by airmail. I'll expect a letter from you tomorrow now.

At 9:30 I went to church. I haven't found anyone to go with me. Three fellows who bunk near me do not belong to the Protestant Church. Two are Catholics and one is a Jew. They are all very nice fellows though and well educated and clean cut. I enjoyed the service quite a bit. I'll enclose the program in this letter. Since you have an hour later than we have here you were in church at the same time. You had church at 10:30 this morning, didn't you? I certainly was glad to be able to "worship" at the same time you did. It made me feel good.

After church, I washed my underwear, socks, handkerchiefs, and towels. We have a washboard and things got very clean. I bought a box of Oxydol[8] at the PX and really scrubbed those things. You've got a very domestic husband when he gets home. Ha! Ha!

This afternoon we changed barracks. All three of those fellows mentioned earlier were separated, we're in different barracks but I've gotten in with other nice men. Heavens, some of these men are smart. Almost all of them are chemists of some sort or pharmacists.

[From the enclosed church program]
Protestant Morning Worship
Hymn-There is a Fountain Filled with Blood-No. 286

---

and they worked around the camp getting $.80 per day. They were most likely used in the kitchens, on ground maintenance and construction projects.
[8] This was a popular laundry soap made by Proctor and Gamble.

Hymn-Almost Persuaded, Now to Believe- No. 341
Hymn- My Faith Looks Up to You- No. 358
Sermon: "Justification By Faith"
[under "Announcements"]

"It is not enough to fight. It is the spirit that we bring to the fight that decides the issue. That type of morals can only come out of the religious nature of a soldier who knows God. I count heavily on that type of man and that type of Army."

[Monday] July 24th

Holy smokes, today I got three letters and a postcard. Boy, that certainly makes things a lot easier. You'll never know how good those letters made me feel. But Ruth, you were a bad girl for biting those nice nails you had. Gosh, that spites me. Now listen to me. You let them grow and don't you dare not let them grow unless you want to make your husband very unhappy. And about that fall you had. You must be more careful. Please, Honey, don't worry about me.

This afternoon we were practicing lining up sights on a sheet with an imitation target. For never looking through a sight of a gun, I did quite well. At 200 yds. on three different sightings, I wasn't more than a 1/4 of an inch apart on any of the 12 sightings.

Boy, I love you. Gee Whiz but I think you're the grandest wife any man ever had. We certainly have a great love for each other.

[Tuesday] July 25th

Gosh, this certainly has been a hectic day for me. For the last few days, another one of those boils has been developing on my "rear". I hadn't written anything about it because it hadn't bothered me that much. Then last night it opened a little. I went to "sick call" this morning and they told me I had to return at 1 PM for the Doctor to lance it. I went back at 1:00 and guess what, they brought me to the Camp Hospital. After arguing with them for about an hour and losing, they made me go to bed. They want to treat me in bed. Boy, am I disgusted, putting you to bed for a boil-they call an abscess. Now I'm missing all the training the other men are getting. They say if it gets better, I'll be out in a day or two. I don't have my toilet articles or anything. The writing paper and pencil I borrowed from the man in the next bed. If you don't hear from me every day it's because I don't have the things to write with.

Now don't worry. I feel fine. The doggone boil doesn't even hurt. It's pretty high up on my rear and I sit in the normal position without noticing anything.

[Wednesday] July 26th

Well, I'm still in the doggone hospital. This morning the doctor lanced the boil that made me grit my teeth a little. I called up my Company Commander and told him where I was. The hospital's all right. You get very good meals. They have books and things to read, but I hate to miss my training.

Gosh, nothing happens in here. I hardly know what to write. I'm about the only fellow here who wants to get out.

How's driving getting along? I see by your letter backing up is improving. I know with a good teacher like your father you'll be one of the best.

Honey, you must get your sleep. Please don't stay awake at night. You mustn't worry about me. And don't think this boil is serious, it's no worse than any of the others I've had. If I'd known they'd bring me to the hospital I'd never have reported to sick call.

P.S. You got your check you told me from the government ($50.00). My gosh, what are you doing with all that money? Ha! Ha! You say we have $1800. Boy, that's good, don't you think, plus about $1000 in bonds. I still have $28 out of the $32 I took along. You certainly don't spend much here.

[Thursday] July 27th (10:30)

My Dearest Darling Wife,

Gosh, I really am disgusted. The doctor is in surgery this morning and can't examine me until this afternoon. Even if he does give me the OK to leave, I'll have to stay here till tomorrow. Boy, that burns me up. I'm missing so many things I should know.

You must excuse me if I don't write much, nothing happens here. This afternoon, after the doctor sees me, I'll write again and let you know what he says. If he won't let me go tomorrow yet, I believe I'll just walk out.

July 27th (5 PM)

I told you I'd write again when I got back from the doctor. He gave me the OK I can leave tomorrow. You check out at 2:30 PM so it'll mean another day wasted. That will mean 3 1/2 days of training I missed. They haven't sent any of my mail up here to the hospital so I haven't gotten any since noon on Tuesday.

When I was over to see the doctor this afternoon, I saw a fellow in a separate room. He had his leg in a big cage with a ray of infrared particles striking it all the time.[9] It looked as though the leg had been practically cut off and they were grafting it together. That certainly was a horrible sight.

---

[9] This was probably an external fixation device for multiple fractures. There was some experimentation with x-ray treatments used to speed up the healing process.

The day goes by and nothing happens here. All I do is walk around, keep hot towels on my rear and look at some magazines.

Does my Dearest Wife still love her hubby? Boy, I hope so because he really loves her.

[Friday] July 28th

Well, I'm back at my company. I got out of the hospital at 2:45. As soon as I got back, I went for my mail. I received 4 letters but he told me he had sent some to the hospital. I didn't get any there so now I'll have to wait until they come back again.

For the last three days, while I was in the hospital, they've been practicing firing. Now without that practice, I've got to go out and shoot for the record. I'll certainly be lucky if I qualify. Wish me luck, I'll need it. I know what I'll do. I'll think of you and how much you're thinking of me and I know I'll make the grade.

I'm so glad to hear that your driving is coming along so well. Honey, you write the nicest letters.

[Saturday] July 29th

Today I got a workout. We got up at 4:15 this morning. Got on our packs and set out for the firing range. It was about a 9 ½-mile walk. Yesterday my First Sergeant said I could fire for the record. Before we left, I told about three of our Lieutenants that I hadn't fired yesterday. One of them shouted at me that I couldn't fire today. The other Lieutenant said I should come along anyway. When I got to the range, they ordered the men to the stations they had the day before. I naturally didn't have a station assigned to me so I went up to a group of officers and told them. Then it happened, they asked the same man who told me I couldn't fire. He remembered me and said, "Weren't you the fellow I told not to fire back in camp?" I said, "Yes Sir." Boy did he "charge" into me before I had a chance to explain. Well, I didn't fire anyway. It doesn't matter too much to me. I don't want to shoot so well anyway yet. I'd like to shoot a good record and stick it under that Lieutenant's nose.

I'll have plenty of time to think of my Honey and how wonderful and darling a wife she is. Boy, she's tops with me. She's a Dear. Don't forget to go to church.

[Sunday] July 30th

It's been only a little over 12hrs. since I wrote you but, gosh, I just feel as though I must write whenever I get a minute to spare. This morning after breakfast I bought a local paper, read it a little, fixed my locker, bed, and such things, and then went to church.

Honey Bunch, (isn't that a nice name for you?) did you notify your employer about that withholding tax? Did you get the car inspected? Be sure and keep practicing at backing. I guess by now you've just about mastered the technique.

Well, my Dear, I've put in 3 full weeks in the Army. All the things we did seem so vivid and clear in my mind that they seem as though they've just happened. In New York we had a grand time; Coney Island, Broadway, Times Square, and Radio City. When this conflict is over and I get back, will we celebrate??

[Monday] July 31st

Gosh Honey, today I was another happy man. I got five letters from Pennsylvania. Boy, Dear, you write the sweetest letters but you seemed a little disappointed in today's letter. You say I don't write enough about myself. Gee whiz, I'm sorry if I write the wrong thing. I'll try and answer all your questions tonight.

This morning they didn't call us to duty till about 8:30. Boy, that seemed strange. Then when they did call us together all we had to do was clean our rifles thoroughly. At 10:30 the fun started. We were told to take our full packs,[10] with mess kit[11] and the like attached, also our rifles and fall in at attention. Then we found we were going on a hike to the Ante Aircraft Firing Range. That was a five-mile hike, through sand and red dirt. The ambulance picked up quite a few who "fell on their faces." It's not so much the distance but the pace they take. It's almost a slow run. When we got to the range, the officer gave us a lecture on Ante Aircraft firing (shooting planes with small firearms). After that we had chow. They bring the food out in trucks and you get your helping in your mess kit. We had roast beef, mashed potatoes, raw cabbage, and creamed cauliflower, and for dessert chocolate cake and iced tea. This afternoon we did our firing. They had moving targets on pulleys and you had to hit them. They traveled at

---

[10] A picture of a Canvas Combat field pack shows it had a two-part design. The smaller pack was for rations, clothes, ammunition and mess kit. The separate Cargo bag, that attached to the bottom, was for extra clothes, shoes and miscellaneous items. The upper part had tabs and loops for attaching a bed roll and other equipment. Some of the items carried included underwear, socks, long johns, sweater, pants, shirt, belt, knit cap, boots, field jacket, rain parka, gloves, blanket, shelter half and personal items that weighed in at about 30 lbs. Then they also carried equipment like a helmet, first aid pouch, canteen, shovel, field bag, k-rations and a hatchet. They also would be carrying their rifle, cleaning kit, cartridge belt, ammunition, bayonet, grenade, gas mask and maybe a radio, battery and binoculars.

[11] The mess kit was metal and fit together with a metal strip. This strip became the handle when opened so you could use it as a skillet over a fire. When closed it would hold your knife, fork and spoon. The lid was divided to use as a dish to put food into.

different speeds. I did rather well. If I were shooting planes instead of targets, I would have hit the planes out of commission with about 90% of my shots. I would have hit the pilot with 50% of my shots. After the firing, the fun really started-the hike back. There were plenty who couldn't take it after being in the hot sun all day. I got back a little tired but none the worse off except for tender soles. With all the sweat that came out of me, I certainly should have lost weight, yet I eat so well I'm afraid I'll get it all back. Ha! Ha!

Dearest, you ask me what a Day Room is. A Day Room is a place where soldiers go to write letters mostly. At our Day Room, they have a ping pong table (which everyone uses to write letters on) and two billiard tables. There are usually about 50 men writing letters and about two or four playing pool.

Abilene is a town of about 25,000 people. They tell me it's a pretty nice town but accommodations are hard to get. If you want to reserve a room at a hotel you must do so about 6 to 8 weeks before and then can only reserve for 3 days. Now I was told the thing to do is to get a room at a private home but you must look for some time to get one. Honey Darling, during these first six weeks they keep you so busy and the restrictions are so narrow that I think it's better to wait for a few weeks.

Honey, you say you don't want me to be any good at shooting. That's the way I feel too when I'm not shooting, but gosh when you get that rifle in your hands you always like to do your best. I guess it's a sense of duty one has.

In all the rain and mud we walked in last week I never once had wet feet. I can't in the world see what makes them so protective. No, my Dear, I don't think my hair is any thinner. I believe it's holding its own. Ha! Ha! My sinus seems to be better, I only had one headache since I'm here that annoyed me to any extent. I believe the weather helps that condition. Honey, you really don't have to worry about me and the "W.A.C."[12] Heavens, I don't see any females of any sort down here. I'll soon forget what a "skirted person" looks like. Ha! Ha! But Honey Dear, I can still see you that Friday night at New Cumberland. You had that new green and white dress on. Boy, you looked so lovely. I'll always have that picture on my mind. Gosh, but I love you.

You asked me again about a picture. Well, my Dear, yesterday afternoon one of the fellows who I learned to know has a camera here. He took my picture and a picture of me and three other fellows. I asked him to have the negatives of those on which I was on so that I could get some made and send them home. He said sure. He still has 3 pictures to take on that film. When they're taken he'll get it developed immediately. I'll send them home as soon as possible. Are you troubled with rats and mice since you want my picture? Ha! Ha!

Gosh, it's getting late. Boy, don't say I don't write enough. Heavens, I've written a book. I hope it's not boring you. Honey, don't worry, for every minute I'm gone we'll have 2 extra minutes of happiness when I get back. Don't forget me but please Honey, you must be happy and gay. Don't be depressed when I'm gone. It'll make me happy to know that there's a smile and gleam you're carrying with you all the time.

Goodnight my Love XXXXX Luke

---

[12] This is related to the Women's Army Auxiliary Corp which was later known at the Women's Army Corp. There was somewhat of a slander campaign against these women due to the muscular nature of their jobs and the jealousy of military wives at home. Many were switchboard operators, mechanics, bakers, drivers and postal clerks.

[Tuesday] August 1st

My Sweetest Dearest Honey Bunch,

Gee whiz Honey, today has given me pain. The officers are really bearing down on this Company. I'm more tired tonight than I was when we went on long hikes. We had one hour of bayonet training (how to kill a man with a bayonet). This afternoon we had classes on first aid and several hours of calisthenics and drill. A soldier in front of me accidentally dropped his rifle and the officer made him run about 1/2 a mile with the rifle above his head. If you'd as much as move your eyes you'd get a bawling out. Tonight after chow, we stood in formation for 1 hour and some 10 minutes. When the officers inspected our hut this morning, they found some that weren't in too good shape. As a result, the whole Company is restricted for an indefinite period.

My Dear if you enjoy my letters half as much as I enjoy yours, you'll feel about 100% better afterward. I see you're enlarging your wardrobe. Ha! Ha! I won't even know you when you come to see me.

I certainly was glad to hear that you managed to get to church on Sunday. That's another thing I like about my wife. In fact, she's tops. I certainly agree with my father when he said I was fortunate to have a wife like you.

[Wednesday] August 2nd

My Sweetest Dearest Darling,

Today I got the good old Reading Times. Boy, it was mighty good to read the news from home. But Honey, I didn't get any letter from you today. I got one from Mother and one from Father though. I guess yours was held up. This afternoon we had two hours of First Aid and two hours of

Hand Grenades.[13] Tomorrow we again go out on the range, this time to throw hand grenades.

We're still restricted to our Company Area. Gosh, my paper is running out as well as my soap. They better lift that restriction soon or else. I did borrow this paper and some blue envelopes from another guy.

Honey Bunch, everyone tells me that you're doing very well at driving. Boy, I'm so glad. You seemed so discouraged sometimes when I took you out. Maybe I wasn't a good teacher? Is that it?

I'm thinking of you every second. I feel so fortunate I have such a fine wife back home.

[Friday] August 4th (6:15 PM)

Yesterday I was so tired I didn't get any letters written so today I'll write two. Will that be alright? Please forgive me.

Yesterday we got the live grenades to throw. We threw from behind a 10-foot wall. The fragments were thrown about 500 ft. at least. I certainly never thought I'd learn to throw a grenade. Just let me have a couple of those in my pocket and I'll fix the doggone Japs. Ha! Ha!

After dinner on the field, which I thought was very good, we hiked back. My feet get so many blisters on them. That's the only thing that troubles me.

---

[13] These were better known as "pineapples" because of the patterned grooved metal body. A ring held the safety pin in place prior to activation. A timed fuse delay ran for approximately 5 seconds after activation where by the operator would lob it at the enemy. The internal content was 2 ounces of TNT, which when detonated would shatter the iron body causing fragments to damage everything within the radius.

August 4th (6:45 PM)

Well, here I go for another letter. Gee whiz Darling I love you.

I'm very glad you went to church at Blandon since your Father had to work. That makes me very proud of you my Dear.

Honey, now don't you forget I most certainly want you to go along to Philadelphia to see your cousin Erma. I wouldn't like it at all if you wouldn't go along. Remember I'm the boss. Ha! Ha!

My Dear, about my "A" book,[14] I'm quite sure I gave that book to my sister. You must ask her for it. However, I don't have any "A 10's" anymore, but starting about the 10th of this month the A1's go into effect. So, you ask Sister for it.

Today we were out on the range again. We had Transition Firing. I did rather well Dear. I don't want to be good just do what they ask me to.

[Saturday] August 5th

This morning we had to stand inspection. Holy Smoke-they (the officers) really were fussy. The Company Commander examined me. He looks at your person, how you're dressed and the like and your bed and your equipment and clothing-how everything's kept. There were about 30 men in our company who were restricted for one thing or another. I believe I forgot to tell you on Thursday our restriction was taken off so I went to the PX and got this paper.

---

[14] This is related to rationing because items needed for the war created short supplies at home. To keep things fair and all get their share the US Office of Price Administration was formed in 1942. Some items rationed were coffee, gasoline, rubber, shoes, sugar, butter, meats and nylons. Ration books and tokens were issued per family. "A" books, for nonessentials, allowed 4 gallons of gas per week, not to be driven for pleasure.

After supper, another soldier and I walked over to the Service Men's Club and got something cold to drink. Then we stopped in at the Camp Library. This man is certainly fine, doesn't smoke or drink. He was a university teacher of Physics in Pittsburg before being drafted.

Boy, he's a smart chap. He asked me to walk along over. He thinks he can talk to me and have me understand what he talks about. He's so deep but very nice.

Tomorrow I'll be going to church again. I still haven't found anybody to go with but I like in a way to worship alone. You'll go too, won't you Honey?

I'm quite sure that I'll get only six weeks of Inf. Basic. Last night they sent some of us over to the Classification Room where they checked each man's record. The way things look now he said we'll be moved to another Company after our 6 weeks and get what he called our Medic Basic. I might be sent out before to some Chemical Laboratory he thought. That would suit me fine especially if it would be closer to Pennsylvania. Ha! Ha!

Tell your parents I asked about them. Are they well? Do you think your Mother would hide from me if I'd come to see her and she had on her trousers? Ha! Ha! You tell her she looks very well in them.

Just wait till we see each other. Will we celebrate?

[Sunday] August 6th

I just had to write. It makes me feel good to write. It seems to bring you closer to me.

My Dear, aren't you going to see any movies lately? You aren't mentioning it to me. Now, I want you to find someone to go with, either my parents or yours or someone, anyone but please honey you must go places. I want you to. Don't worry, I know you'll behave all right.

Did you see the Doctor? I think you should see him anyway and tell him about everything. Tell him that we want one badly and that he should find the trouble so that when I come back, we can get busy. Ha! Ha! Ha! I'm getting doggone anxious for a child myself.

Honey, Dear, I love you so very, very much. You're such a grand wife. Gosh, we're going to be so very happy together, aren't we? My Darling, you mustn't think of those times we had that weren't so pleasant. Those we'll just forget. They're gone forever. All we'll think of now is the pleasant times we've spent together and those we're going to spend. We love each other so very much, don't we honey?

I'll get paid around the 10th of this month. I still have about 23 dollars.

[Monday] August 7th

My Sweetest Dearest Honey Darling,

Boy is that a salutation!! I could add a lot more adjectives because there are so many that fit my dear. She's the dearest thing (how do you like being called a thing) in the world.

I got 4 letters today, the Reading Times, and I got that certificate for that course I took at Albright.

Gee whiz darling I'm glad you got letters. I can't see why you don't get a letter a day. I write one every day.

This morning we got up at 5 AM. We were issued carbines.[15] They fire the same caliber shell as the rifle we have but are much lighter in weight. Then we marched out to the range. If I was shooting a man instead of targets, I would have shot him on every shot. After I was finished a lieutenant borrowed my weapon and fired. Heavens, I did much better

---

[15]The M1 carbine was the standard weapon. It fired 8 rounds per clip and still is used by drill teams and military honor guards.

than he did and me never shooting a gun before in my life. It must be what they call beginners luck. Ha! Ha!

Honey Darling you mustn't worry about me. I shoot well, that doesn't mean anything in particular. I'm still better, I would think at my work. If they want me as a gunner, OK I'll do my best but I'm not worried about that. I feel quite sure I'm definitely in the Medical Corps.

I don't know what's holding up those pretzels Mother sent; I'm tasting them in my mouth for such a long time.

Honey Bunch, when I get to Abilene, I'm going to the Travelers Aid.[16] I hear they have the names of people who will take in soldier's wives, that is have an extra room or two and there will be no limit on how long you can stay. How would you like that?

Good night my Dear.

[Tuesday] August 8th

Today we had a little of everything. This morning we had two hours of first aid, one hour of Defense Against Mechanical Attacks, and one hour of drill.

So now they're raising cats over at home. Ha! Ha! Small kittens are so cute, aren't they?

Honey, by your letter of the 4th, you hint that you were going to take your test yesterday. Did You?

I'm glad to hear that you received such a fine and expensive prize from your employer. It makes me doubly proud of my darling. You must have done a grand job when you were a manager.

---

[16] The National Travelers Aide Association was a movement started in 1851 helping travelers move west from St. Louis, Missouri. Early in the 20th century the idea moved to several large cities and became very helpful during World War II, especially with women meeting up with their significant others while at military training bases.

Yes, my Dear, I think you should make an appointment with the Doctor. I'd tell him to get busy and find out the trouble. We want to start on our family any day now. I'll "f--k" you every day until something happens. We'll get there don't worry.

One learns to appreciate good people like yourself when one can't share life with them for a while.

[Wednesday] August 9th

Hello Sweet Stuff!!

This morning we had an hour on Malaria[17] and insects.

This noon for dessert we had watermelon. Boy, it's the first I've had for some time and it was so very good.

Last night there was a USO[18] show in our Company Theater and guess who was in it- Katherine Behney and her girls from Reading, Pa.-you know who I mean? She has a dance studio in Reading. I went down and just got there when they were doing their last number. I understand they are touring the country with this show.

[Thursday] August 10th

Today was a big day for us soldiers. Payday!! I received in cold cash $21.40, from July 10th to August 1st. I get $6.70 a month off for insurance. I'm going to start saving for a furlough or maybe even send some home.

Today we had an hour of compass and map reading and an hour on how to prepare a full pack. I guess by next week

---

[17] There wasn't any vaccine for Malaria which is mosquito borne. Soldiers could get Atabrine to treat it if symptoms started.

[18] The United Service Organizations, started in 1941, were not government agencies but maintained through private contributions from individuals and corporations. They organized camp shows in the US and overseas to lift the spirits of the troops and make them feel more at home.

we'll be going on some long hikes and pitch tents and stay out for a few nights. I certainly hope I'll be able to write every day.

I want to say I'm very well pleased you passed your driver's test.

When the sweat rolls off of me and the job ahead seem so hard, I just think of my Dear and everything comes out fine.

[Friday] August 11th

Gosh, my Dear, I've been so very busy tonight I have to write this in the latrine for the lights are out in the barracks. Tomorrow morning, we have an inspection on the field, and boy they're really going to be strict. There are so many things that have to be "just" so or else.

This afternoon we were out on the camouflage range. We were taught all about how to set up camouflage and when etc. Next week when we go on bivouac, we'll have to know these things.

No, my Honey, I'm not mad because you didn't tell me when you were taking your test. Gee whiz I'm glad you passed.

[Saturday] August 12th

Well, still another kind of paper. I'm getting various kinds of paper, am I not?

Today was another "lulu". This morning we had a field inspection. We were standing at attention while the commanding officer came along. When he came in front of you, you had to come to "inspection arms" with your rifle and he checked it. I really looked like a soldier and felt like one.

Gosh Honey, today completed four weeks of my basic training and I'm not one bit sorry. I never thought a man could be taught so much in so short a time.

Well, my Dear, you drove to Leesport alone you tell me. I guess you feel pretty proud of yourself, don't you?

My Dearest don't you think I've acquired any bad habits!! Absolutely haven't. Many a time the beverage at our meal is coffee but I still haven't touched a drop of it and I don't intend to. And I haven't smoked or drunk a bit. That's God's truth, believe me.

[Sunday] August 13th

Hello Honey Bunch!! So, you're jealous of my parents since I used that name in their letter. Ha! Ha! Well, guess I can't do that anymore, how about it?

I was in church again this morning. It's the one thing one does in a week that comes close to what one does at home on a Sunday.

At your leisure, you can send me some Army socks and some undershirts. Washing takes so much time in the evenings that I can hardly get my two letters in. If I'd have some extra socks and undershirts, I'd be able to go for a long time without washing. You and Mother can get together on the whole thing, I guess.

Say my Darling, are you waxing the car? You said you were going to start last week. Gosh my Dear, you want to keep our car shined up, don't you? Do you think you're strong enough to wash it? Ha! Ha!

Don't you ever think that you're writing too much. You could write a lot more if you want to.

My Dear, it doesn't matter to me at all what you do with your hair. I like them short or long. You know me, honey. I know you're swell either way. You're so very beautiful.

[Monday] August 14th

Today I was extra lucky. I received 5 letters, 3 boxes and 2 papers. One was from Carpenter Steel telling me they'll pay $1000 of my policy when I return after the war. I received your box of Caramel Corn, another box of Billy's Pretzels, and a box of food from Mother and Grandma. I think I'll start a "snack lunch cafeteria" in my barracks. Ha! Ha! When I walked into the barracks with all my packages and mail, they were all amazed. I'm so thankful when I think how wonderful you are that it almost makes tears of happiness come to my eyes.

This morning we had an hour of calisthenics and boy they were tough. The officers said they wanted to get us in shape for the "Obstacle Course" which they said was a real tough one. Afterward, we had a few hours on Preparations of Fox Holes and Trenches. Then we witnessed a parade. We'll have to participate in the next one. The whole regiment parades in front of the reviewing stand with the officers of the Camp, from the General on down, in the stands. Boy, that makes you feel like a soldier.

You know we have some Prisoners of War here, about 6,000. Today I saw quite a few of them. They were putting new tin chimneys on our barracks. Boy, they were big husky men and they looked terribly strong. They were full-blooded Germans.

Honey, you haven't heard from Howard yet, have you? Now, remember when you hear please let me know. I'm so anxious to know. I think about him so much lately, and today when I saw these men. I was wondering what he was doing. I'm quite sure he's OK. All we can do is wait to hear from him. I was told here that the Germans, especially lately, are treating our men very well because they know they're licked and by treating our captured men well they hope to get better peace terms from our Armies. So, we really can be thankful for that. That sounds very logical too.

[Tuesday] August 15th

This morning we had three hours of laying "mines". We had to lay a whole minefield, dig them in the earth and then root them up and collect them again. After a long day, I had to stand guard for two hours from 6:30 to 8:30 PM. I had to walk my post for two hours and one can't stop walking either or he'll really get the devil.

Tonight after 8:30 I received a small shovel to build my fox home. On Thursday night I'll be away from camp on a hike so I'm not sure whether I'll be able to write. You understand, don't you Honey Bunch?

Honey, you don't gossip. I just love to read your letters. Please don't ever cut them short.

Honey, as of yet I haven't used my money belt. I've used my purse exclusively. I've always kept it in my pocket. Nothing has been taken from me yet.

I hope you miss me as much as I miss you. Boy, will that be a happy day when I'll again hold you in my arms.

P.S. I'm eligible to go to Officer's Candidate School after my basic. That is the school where you become an Officer. I'm qualified because of my training and my grades. I was told that my grades put me in the "superior" group. I don't know yet what I'll do.

[Saturday] August 19th

Gosh, my Dear, I missed three days in writing. It's terrible, I know, but I just was too busy to write. On Wednesday night I wrote a small note, only that night we had to pack our field packs and get ready for our trip. At 2:30 AM we got up and finished packing. At 3:30 we started our march with full packs. At 7:30 we reached our destination. That was a terrific pace. Even the commanding officer admitted that it was too fast a pace. Quite a few men fell over unconscious. Their minds, the doctor said, were absolutely blank. Plenty of men could not stand it. On the way, we had a practice air raid drill. We walked a half-hour with our gas masks on.

Well, when we finally reached our "area" we had to pitch our tents and dig our fox hole. It took us about 3 hours to dig the hole. It was almost solid rock and all we had was a small shovel.

After lunch, we had practice on "Extended Order Drill". That is practicing going into enemy-held territory. I was a rifleman on our squad. We practiced entering a wood held by the enemy.

That night rain came up and boy did we get wet. I slept that night on a blanket with all my clothing on. Surprising as it may seem I slept very well, even though I was pretty well soaked.

On Friday morning we probed a whole minefield; that is, we probed the ground for mines on hands and knees.

We arrived back at Camp at 8 that night and the next morning had a rigid field inspection. Gosh, that kept me stepping.

This morning after inspection we had two hours of lecture on "Booby Traps" and the secrets of military operations.

I love you more than you can ever guess. Gosh, my Dear, I miss your loving smile and lovely welcome expressions, your kindness, and your hospitality.

[August] 19th (card sent for their 5th Wedding Anniversary)

Gee whiz, my Dear, I just couldn't find a suitable card. This was the nearest thing I could find. Please accept it in the spirit with which it's sent. Happy Anniversary Dear. When I get back, I'll get that gift you always wanted. Remember I just can't buy that here. You'll understand, won't you?

[Sunday] August 20th

Hello Honeybunch and Darling Sugar-Pie,

Well, here's another Sunday rolling around and as far as I'm concerned, every day could be Sunday. It's the easiest day I have.

As you know on Wednesday it's our Fifth Wedding Anniversary. Gosh, it's just too bad we won't be able to celebrate our anniversary together but such is the way of life. I can only say this: August 23, 1939, turned out to be the luckiest day in my life, for on that day I married absolutely the finest lady in God's World.

Honey, you said I used an ugly word in my letter. Well honey you didn't use that same word but you inferred that same thing in your letter. So, you'll demand three a night! Well, I'm sure I can take it. The thing is, I doubt very much whether you can. Ha! Ha! And don't think you can ever wear me out. That's an impossibility. Remember that.

Yes, my Dear, we didn't get to spend our vacation in Wildwood did we? They'll always be a "new day dawning" so we have much to look forward to. Don't worry, my Dear, we'll spend many a fine vacation together. We'll have such grand fun.

Yes, I love you as much as ever. If I can grow fonder of you I am. I love you now as much as is humanly possible and yet I never dreamed I could miss you and long for a person as I do you.

Dearest, you take account of what you spend on my parent's gifts and please for my sake let me know. You're so thoughtful about getting them. I'll try and get cards for them if I can get into Abilene today.

They say you must wait about an hour to an hour and a half for a bus to get in.

You make fun of my marching at home but let me tell you this, I was never corrected or told how to march here. In fact, I was pointed out as an example of correct marching. So that's one-time dear I wasn't wrong. Ha! Ha!

Honey, as soon as I'm sure I'll be here for eleven weeks after my six are over I'll inquire immediately as to your living here and let you know all the details. There are so many reports of what might happen to some of us that it would be foolish to make plans and then having to break them.

Honey Darling, you sealed one of your letters with a kiss. Gosh, my dear, you do the grandest things.

You tell me Donald Kauffman and Bruce High were wounded. That's just too bad. My Mother also wrote me that Frank Kunkle was killed in France. His father drives Yoder's meat truck. He was a fine fellow. He played in the Centerport Band. It's just too bad that such things have to happen.

[Monday] August 21st

Gosh Honey, I'm a happy person tonight. Of course, before the night's over I'll be pretty tired. At 7:30 PM we're hiking to the "Infiltration Course" where we'll have machine gun bullets flying over our heads and we have to crawl and go under barbed wire fences. Boy, that'll be something.

I got four fine Anniversary cards, one from you, one from Mother, one from Mother-in-Law, and one from Grandmother. Gosh, they were fine cards. I also got three dollars in cash.

This morning I had an hour of Physical Conditioning, an hour on Scouting and the use of compasses, an hour on how to creep and crawl, and then an hour of actual practice on the infiltration course. This afternoon we had two hours of detection of various planes.

Honey, I'm so thankful for our great lives. It gives one the spirit to carry despite seemingly unobtainable obstacles.

[Tuesday] August 22nd

Gee whiz, it's 10 PM and I'm just getting started with my letter writing. Holy Smokes I've been busy again today. One hardly gets a moment to himself this week.

Honey, that card I received from you was so very nice. I only wish I could have selected such a fine card. Honey, my Dear, I just couldn't find any. I went to almost every store I could find and they just didn't have the kind I would have liked. Honey Bunch, I hope you received the flowers I sent you.

Honey, I was called up to the Dispensary at 10:15 PM for a profile test. They gave me a general check-up. They marked me down on my feet and heartbeat. I have no idea what it all means. Now I'm writing in the Latrine finishing this letter. I'm bound to write tonight if I'm up all night.

I stood guard mount from 6:30- 8:30 PM with my rifle. Gosh, a man gets tired of walking for two hours with his rifle.

Honey, I don't know at all where I'll go or what I'll do after this week. I've heard so many rumors I don't know what to think.

[Wednesday] August 23rd

I'm so sorry I can't get a decent letter in anymore. I know I'll be moved at the end of the week even if it is within Camp Barkeley. We'll either move somewhere else in Barkeley or ship out of the camp. I don't know what will happen.

I got a very nice letter from Mother. Say, is the Infantile Paralysis[19] epidemic hitting Leesport? What in the world is happening to that community since I left?

This afternoon we had lectures by a Catholic Priest, a Rabbi, and a Protestant Minister. They talked of the unity of race and religion, not to have hatred toward one another.

[Thursday] August 24th

Something must have happened with Uncle Sam's mail service. Today is the second straight day I didn't get a letter from my darling. Is she getting to be too busy to write? Ha! Ha! No, my dear, I know that it must be the mail that's at fault, not my wife.

Today I received the box of clothing etc. that you and Mother sent. Gosh, everything was just fine.

Honey Darling, today the fellow that took my picture got his pictures back. I saw the one of myself. It's not too good but it will have to pass. He gave me the negative so I'll enclose it in this letter and you can get all made you want. Probably Mother and Father would like one.

At 7:45 tonight we'll have to fall in formation. We're going on a 4-mile hike and then we'll have a night problem on Scouting and Patrolling. We'll get back at almost 12:30 AM. We'll be starting on another hike at 5:30 tomorrow morning so you see we're kept mighty busy.

On Saturday night we're shipping out of this Company and Battalion. So, you see my address will be changed. As soon as I get it, I'll send it on to you immediately.

---

[19] This was the Poliovirus which was highly contagious, transmitted by contaminated food and water. The most serious epidemics occurred in the 1940's and 1950's. Jonas Salk tested his vaccine in 1952 and mass vaccinations were promoted by the March of Dimes in 1957.

What happened to that front tire? You tell me you believe the tube is bad. Well, that is the tire I probably put the old tube back in when I got the new tires. If the tube is bad you can buy another one. You know they are not rationed anymore.

I hear you were up at Leesport on Sunday for dinner and that you won the one game of Rook that was played. Pretty good, aren't you? Ha! Ha!

Say, my Dear, you never sent me any of those pictures we took before I left for the Army. How about sending at least two or three of your poses of us together? But wait until I'm placed again.

[Friday] August 25th (10:15 PM)

Gosh my Dear I feel good tonight. In the first place, I received five letters, 3 from my dear Honey Bunch and 2 from Mother.

As you can see the hour is late again. I'm sitting outside on the walk under a lamp to write this letter. Lights just went out and I've been busy all day and night. Tomorrow morning, we have an inspection and since we hand in our rifles tomorrow, they're really going to be exact. I also had to wash my leggings[20] and cartridge belt. Today we hiked about 12 miles, did scouting and patrolling, and set "booby traps".

I'm glad Allen gave you a new tube. I'm sure he'll treat you right. He always did me, anyway.

Honey, if I stay in Camp Barkeley I'll get to Abilene the first chance I get to look into getting a room. Believe me, I will.

---

[20] These were pieces of canvas with either hooks or buckles worn over the top of boots to keep dirt, bugs etc. out. They began to disappear when higher top boots were issued.

Gee whiz, Honey, we'll have to start on our family. You know what, I think I want about three children. My wife will make a very good mother. She can't miss because she's such a very good wife.

Medical Basic Training at Camp Barkeley

[Saturday] August 26th

Well, my Dear, I've moved and I'm still at Camp Barkeley believe it or not. It's entirely in another part of Camp, however about 3 miles from where I was. It's in the 56th Company C. We're allowed to have our lights on until 10:00. We must be in our beds at 10:30 PM.

The place here, I think I'll like better than the old one. There's grass growing around here which wasn't true at our old company, and the barracks are quite a bit nicer. We'll get quite a few marches and drills which will consist of carrying other men (representing wounded soldiers). I also think there will be a lot of classwork and lectures.

Tomorrow we'll be processed, that is we'll be classified into various groups according to our abilities and the like.

[Sunday] August 27th

How are the gladiolas that I sent you getting along? Do those flowers last very long? Do you like that kind of flower? -or do you like roses better? I thought I'd order some other kind for a change. I certainly hope that you liked them.

This morning I didn't get to church. I found out that we have quite a nice chapel that our Company is attached to but this morning we must remain in our huts to receive various orders. As a result, I can't get to church.

Tomorrow I start my Medical Basic. How long it'll be I do not know. It won't be more than 11 weeks. They might ship me out before then, however. My Dear, I asked our Corporal if we'd be able to get into Abilene this afternoon and he said he was afraid not.

If anything, the food seems even better. At our old company, we were served in a cafeteria manner. Here everything is right on the table. If you want any more you just go back to the kitchen and fill up.

We're just in the midst of a mild thunderstorm. The sky is all black and overcast. It's thundering too. How is the weather in Berks these days? I hope your heatwave has concluded?

Well, my Dear, it's been seven full weeks now that I've been in the service. Gee whiz, it seems like such a long time. I'm certainly lucky to be able to have such wonderful memories of what my life was like before I entered the Army and such pleasant thoughts of what it's going to be like after this conflict is over.

Thoughts such as that, make up for all the tough things one goes through in the Army. It gives one faith and courage to fight on despite all the difficulties that may come up. I'm sure that I never thought I'd be able to do all I did but now that it's over, I'm none the worse off, in fact, it makes a fellow feel as though no obstacle is too big for him now. It gives a man loads of confidence.

Honey Darling, I just love and love and love you. Always love me real, real much.

[Monday] August 28th

Hello, my Dear. How's everything? Is my honey still in love with me? I certainly hope so.

We had rain all day today. The place was quite muddy. It's funny in Texas you either have dust or mud, but mostly dust.

This morning we had an hour of speeches by our Company and Battalion officers, an hour of the Care of Casualties, and an hour on the Treatment of Gas Victims.[21] I believe that we'll have very much technical training here. They'll teach us a lot about the physiology and anatomy of the human body, how to aid and care for the wounded. However, we're due for quite a few marches also. We'll get quite a few examinations I hear. The first one we're having on Wednesday already. We have to study in the evenings now just like when we were in school and college. Ha! Ha!

Honey, you can't possibly enjoy my letters any more than I do yours. Boy, I can hardly wait until I get to mail call and hear my name called. Yes, last week I was hoping that that week would soon be over, now I'm hoping that the next eleven weeks will be over in a hurry.

Yes, we were a little nervous on August 23, 1939, weren't we? I can still see my honey as though it were yesterday. She had on blue shoes and a blue skirt and blouse. My, but she was so beautiful. Gosh, but I'm very lucky to have such a grand and glorious wife. I only hope that I'm worthy of her. I hope I am.

Oodles of Love and Kisses

[Tuesday] August 29th

This morning we had four straight hours of lectures, two hours of Materia Medica[22] and Pharmacy, an hour of Emergency and Care of Casualties, and an hour of Field

---

[21] Chemical warfare was used during World War I to disable troops. The chemicals could remain active for several days. World War II troops were taught about smells and appearance of gases but very little chemical warfare was used on either side.

[22] This is a Latin term for knowledge related to medical healing.

Sanitation.[23]I wouldn't mind this sort of work but those hikes we get are not exactly "up my alley". We have a 9-mile march on Thursday morning.

Yes, the man that taught at Duquesne University[24] is still in the same group that I'm in. Probably got the same qualifications for being here that I have.

Gosh, my Dear, I'm proud of you. You really are very smart to clean and wax the car. I'll bet she shines. Honey Dear, that was sweet of you. I'm very glad to hear that you take pride in our car. But it's quite a bit of work, isn't it? It makes one pretty tired. It's so doggone much rubbing to it, isn't it? But after it's all done, one feels proud of the work he's done. The car looks like new, doesn't it? Gosh, I wish I could see how it looks.

Yes, we would surely have gone to see Brooklyn play Carpenter Steel. We always enjoyed baseball games, didn't we?

I guess the flowers are pretty faded by this time. But I'm sure the thought behind them will never fade.

[Wednesday] August 30th

This morning we had four straight hours of lectures and an hour of bandaging. Yes, they teach you how to bandage any kind of wound. We had another hour of anatomy and physiology, pharmacy, and Transportation of the Sick and Wounded.

---

[23] These courses taught the soldier personal hygiene, placement and upkeep of latrines, water purification, use of repellants and food preparation. It also emphasized the need to report to sick call at the first sign of illness, complying with set rules and how individual health has an effect on the entire unit.

[24] A Catholic school founded in 1878 located in Pittsburg, Pa.

We had an examination from 4-5 PM. We answered all the questions after the exam and I had them all right. I guessed quite a few of them. Ha! Ha!

[Thursday] August 31st

Well, this morning we had our hike. We made it in a very good time. They claim that the Medical Soldier[25] does more walking than any soldier of any other branch. We'll have to average 7 miles per hour by the end of our training.

Honey Dear, things still seem very unsettled but I'm going ahead and make arrangements for your coming down. I was told that many new men are going to Technician School in about two weeks. Previously I was told that I probably wouldn't have to go to school, that I was already classified as a Chemical Technician. However, they need quite a few Pharmacists right now and I was told that my qualifications are just right for me to go to Pharmacy School and become a Pharmacist Technician as well as a Chemical Technician. Time is approaching when I'll have to decide about going to O.C.S. I don't know what I'd rather do. What I'm afraid of is that if you're an officer, you'll have a harder time getting out of the service after the war. Of course, maybe there'd be lots of chances of getting a good position if you're an officer after the war is over.

---

[25] Some of the medics were conscientious objectors, did not carry a weapon and were looked down upon by some, but any medic in combat was loved and respected. By wearing a Red Cross symbol on their helmet and arm band it made them targets under fire. They provided care under fire, retrieved the wounded, provided medical care in the absence of a physician and continued care and monitoring of troop health in camp.

[Friday] September 1st

I hope that picture I sent you isn't too bad. It's the best you can get I guess with a "face like mine". Ha! Ha!

Today was such a very hard day. We had two hours of bandaging and two hours of Organization of BM Equipment this morning. This afternoon we had two hours of learning how to make knots and lashes and two hours of Mass Athletics.

Tomorrow we have an inspection and they say you really must be right or else. Your person must be just right, even your belt must overlap just 1/2 inch. No more or less.

No, my dear, unless things change, I won't be using a rifle anymore unless I'm sent overseas. Even then I doubt that I'll be upfront. Unless they have a shortage of "gunners" I'm safe. My record with the rifle and carbine was quite good but as things stand now, I've been definitely assigned Medical Corps.

[Saturday] September 2nd

My Dearest Honey Snookums,

There's a new salutation for you my dear. How do you like it? Today, my Dear, I was somewhat disappointed. I didn't receive a letter from my wife, in fact, I didn't receive a letter from anybody; no mail at all.

This noon we had a very good dinner. It consisted of turkey, mashed potatoes, peas, salad, lemonade, and ice cream. It was one of the best meals I've had in the Army. Of course, it still doesn't come up to the cooking I get at Mother Kunkleman's or Mother Snyder's place. Theirs is tops.

Tomorrow or Tuesday I think I'll get my first chance in the kitchen. I believe I'll draw K.P. one of those days. I've been in almost eight weeks and haven't been on detail work except for guard duty two nights.

Gosh, my Dear, I'm at a loss to know what to do. I'd hate to make arrangements for you to come down here and then have to move out at about the same time that you'd come. I believe the fare is about $80 by train round trip. It's quite a bit cheaper by bus though.

[Sunday] September 3rd

Today was quite a nerve "racking" day for me. In the first place, we had our inspection at 1 PM and they are tough. Also, every morning they have a "hut" inspection. On Friday they gave everybody in our hut a Demerit. My towel was hung on the hanger the wrong way. I never knew before there was a particular way to hang it. I was determined that was the last demerit I was going to get.

In the afternoon another group of officers went through the hut again. When we came back to our hut 80% of the beds were torn up. Mine was intact. Boy, that made me feel good. There aren't more than a few in the Company of 225 that have only one Demerit.

I hear there's a 16-mile hike in store for us.

Honey, why don't you go to see some movies? Please seek some entertainment. I believe you should tell the manager only when I find out definitely when you will come. I have a notion to go to my Commanding Officer and see if he knows just what's in store for me.

Yes, my Dear, I got a haircut last Monday. No boils, no headaches, no foot trouble, or sinus. Yes, Honey, I have everything I need right now.

[Monday] September 4th

I received my ballot to vote on Election Day, November 7th. It's a ballot just like you people will get only it's marked "Military Ballot".

Honey, you certainly are exaggerating with regards to that picture. It's impossible, especially a snapshot to look as good as you say that one does. However, I'm glad that it made you feel good. Let me know how the enlargements came out.

(taken from Sunday church program)
Chapel No. 3 Camp Barkeley, Texas
Col. Taylor E. Darby Commanding
Hymn- All Hail the Power of Jesus Name
Hymn- My Jesus I Love Thee
Sermon- "The Comforter"
Hymn- Take the Name of Jesus with You
(after Benediction)
Hymn-God Bless America
[Tuesday] September 5th
Honey, the mail must have gone screwy again. I didn't hear from you today.

Tomorrow I'm on K.P. from 5 AM to 8 PM and tonight from 6 to 8 PM. I had to go in already and start preparing for tomorrow.

This afternoon we had an 8-mile march with full field packs, our gas masks plus our medical kits.[26] I wish you could have seen me with all that stuff on. I really looked like a "fighting" soldier. Ha! Ha!

How is the gas situation? Do you have enough for driving? You only have an "A" book, don't you? Honey, if

---

[26] This was a canvas bag that could be attached to a waist belt or shoulder strap. The contents changed as technology during the war changed. It contained several different kinds of bandages, scissors, tweezers, iodine swabs, medical tags to ID the wounded or dead, adhesive tape, thermometer, safety pins, tourniquets, aromatic spirits, scalpel, vaseline gauze, hypodermic needles and syringes and morphine for pain. There was also burn kits, nitroglycerine for cardiac, surgical needles, sulfa powder and much more.

you want to, why don't you use the car to go to Reading to work? Of course, you'd have to apply for supplementary gas. If you prefer the bus it's all right.

Yes, those flowers lasted real long. I don't know exactly how gladiolas look but I can remember that they are rather nice flowers. Did you forget to send me some of those snapshots that we took? I want some of yours (with you alone or with you and someone else).

Honey, they've started to ship some men to school. Small groups will leave for the next two weeks. Gee Whiz, I wish I knew what the future holds.

Honey Bunch, do you love your husband yet? Sometimes I believe that you're sorry you married me. By the way you write, you consider yourself lucky to have "captured" me.

[Wednesday] September 6th

Boy, was I lucky today! Received two letters from my darling wife and was glad to receive that one with the pictures in it. Boy, I'm glad to see those faces. My wife looks so very beautiful. I was so proud of them. I showed them to my few friends and they all said I was really lucky to get such a beautiful woman.

Today I was on K.P. We got off at 7 PM instead of 8. I had mentioned we had to scrub and mop the whole kitchen and all the tables after every meal. You can't imagine how much work there is to make a meal for about 250 men.

Gee Whiz, my Dear, you mustn't think I'd scold you for getting a dent in the fender. I don't believe it was even your fault the way you say. Charles is a little slow and far from being alert. You just pay for it, but use some of our money. Don't use your money. No Darling, you just keep driving. Don't let a little dent make you nervous.

[Friday] September 8th

Last night we had a march from 7 PM to 10 PM. We covered about 10 1/2 miles. We were supposed to make it in 4 hours and they got back 55 minutes ahead of schedule. We carried about 55 lbs. on our backs. I never thought I'd be able to walk so fast and so long but I'm none the worse off for it. I feel good.

Yesterday afternoon we had two hours of the Nomenclature and Organization of Medical Equipment.

Today we had two hours of keeping Medical Records of the Wounded Men from the front lines until they reach hospitals in the U.S. A detailed record is kept from the time they're wounded even when they are given as much as a cup of coffee.

After supper, we scrubbed our barracks for inspection tomorrow. The rest of the evening we are free for a change so I just must write to my loved ones.

I certainly am glad to hear Sister is home. I know everybody up home feels much better now that she came back. I hear that she isn't too well. Mother writes that the Doctor was there and that he ordered complete rest for her. I believe she's suffering from nervous exhaustion.

No, my Dear, I'm absolutely not angry at you at all for getting that dent in the fender. That happens to the best of drivers. You mustn't let that worry you or unnerve you.

No Honey, this man from Duquesne University is not married, but I believe the next thing to it. He's my age, in fact, a little older. He was 26 on Monday so he's a few months older than I am. Yes, I know a few men who have their wives living in Abilene. None, however, are from Pennsylvania. They are all from closer to Texas. Gee Whiz, I'm anxious to have you come down here as you are to come but things are so uncertain. In the next two weeks, I may not even be in Texas anymore.

Honey, I certainly do not look any more handsome now than I did before July 10th. I might be thinner but I'm certainly as ugly looking as ever. Ha! Ha!

[Saturday] September 9th

At 3 PM we had our Personal Inspection. Holy Smokes, was the Inspection officer tough. He "gigged" about 90% of the men. He caught most soldiers by asking them one or more of the general orders. These are orders, every soldier should know. I knew the one he asked me luckily enough. They are really getting tough with us medical soldiers.

Honey, this noon they called about 20 men's names out, and by 5 PM were out of camp already, probably going to Technician School. By gosh honey, what shall we do? I'm at a loss to know what will happen. Even our Company Officers have no idea who will ship out. They wait for orders from Regimental Headquarters.

My Dear, do you think it's wise for you to come down? I might be here 9 weeks or more and I might leave any day at any hour. Now listen, if you think it's safe or you want to run the risk I'll look after a room right away and let you know.

In the group that left today was that chap from Emmaus, Pa. Now he was just a college student. He probably will get more schooling. The University professor is still here.

Mother writes that the doctor wants to inject some vitamin solution into Sister to aid her in gaining strength. I certainly hope she gains strength in a hurry. She's probably terribly thin.

I'm sort of proud of myself. I went through this whole past week without getting a single demerit and from what I hear that was true with only a few men.

P.S. Darling you didn't forget that Mother's birthday is on September 13th? Please write when your parent's birthdays are and anniversary.

[Sunday] September 10th

You have 8:05 now and I guess you're in church right now. Rev. Stoudt has that dedication program for those hymn books, doesn't he? I certainly wish I was home and able to worship with my darling. Everything that I do with my wife seems so much more real than when we're alone.

Gosh Honey, you wrote such a nice long letter. I could read your letters every minute of the day. Honey, you seemed rather heart-broken since you still didn't hear anything definite from me. I realize it, my Dear, but I actually don't know what to do. This noon they came running through the huts and called out more names. At 3 PM they left for points unknown. They yelled Snyder this noon and I thought I was on my way but it was the other "Snyder". They tell you to be ready in a few hours.

I went to church at 10 AM. Today I believe was the finest church service I've ever attended in the Army. We also had Holy Communion and it was very impressive. The bread and wine were passed out to you at your seat and then the Chaplain and the members all took the elements together. Gee whiz, it was so impressive and he preached a very fine sermon.

This afternoon I washed some clothes for about two hours. At 3 PM the University professor came into my hut and asked if I'd go along up to the chapel. He asked the chaplain for the keys to the electric organ and he played for about an hour. Gee, the music sounded very good. He played practically all church hymns and organ preludes. He played the organ in his church at Pittsburg. He's a very fine man. I never hear him use a single curse word. He doesn't smoke or drink. He certainly hopes either of us won't be separated. He thinks I have so much in common with him. I guess he can talk things to me that others wouldn't understand. And I don't understand some of the things he says myself.

There isn't a soul in the hut here right now. They're all gone away, I guess. It's nice to be alone though, I can think so much better and recall so many fine thoughts of our past life and our happy future life.

I'm glad to hear you got your $50 check. Yes, honey, you didn't tell me it when you got the check but I'll gladly forgive my dear. She just forgot it; anybody can forget things. You're forgiven my honey. Now you use that money if you need anything.

Yes, my eyes are still blue and my muscles are getting pretty tough and I still have hair on my chest. Ha! Ha! Ha!

Honey, I'm enclosing some pictures that were taken at the same time that one was that you have of me. On the back of one of them, I'll tell you who the men are.

[Monday] September 11th

I was very lucky today again. I received 4 letters and two papers. Boy, that American League race is close between New York, Detroit, and St. Louis. Those games are getting interesting. I'm rooting for the St. Louis Browns. The World Series would then be a "city series" between the Cards and Browns.

This morning we had two hours of heavy Tent Pitching.

Just got back from Mass Athletics. I was playing softball. That stuff is all right during regular hours but I certainly am not fond of having it after the evening meal. It takes up so much of one's evening.

I see by the schedule of the week that we have three exams in the latter part of the week. Yes, I take notes in almost every class. They throw so much at you that if you don't take it down, you'll not be able to remember it all.

Honey Bunch, a Battalion is bigger than a Company. In every Battalion there are four Co's-Co A, B, C, D. Three Battalions make up a Regiment. Two Regiments make up a Division and so on up. Each Company is divided into Platoons. I'm in the 4th Platoon of Company C which is part of the 56th Battalion which is a part of the 12th Regiment. Do you understand now?

[Tuesday] September 12th

My Sweetest Honey Lamb,

I always look forward to mail call.

Well, my Dear, today was another big day for me. It was time for the "soldier" to get paid. I received $21.10 for August. Gosh, I feel like a rich man with all that money in my pocket. I believe if I can get money on hand for a furlough, I'll get a "bond" a month.

You know there are special bonds[27] for soldiers. They are $10 bonds. You pay $7.50 and receive a $10 maturity value. Yes, this is one bright day for the soldiers when they receive their few cents. Ha!

This evening after chow I went to the PX and got a haircut. Gosh, but you must even wait in line for a haircut. When I finally got on the chair and the barber started to cut my hair, he asked me if I wanted a treatment for my hair (that is to bring some hair back). I said no that I tried so much and

---

[27] To help cover the expenses of the war the US Treasury encouraged Americans to purchase E bonds. A $25 bond would be worth $18.75 and in 10 years when cashed in would be worth full value.

it never helped. Then he went on to tell me how this tonic worked, that it just came out a few months ago and has worked very well. I told him I'd think it over until I came in the next time. He probably wanted to sell me some cheap stuff and charge me an exorbitant fee.

Gosh, but I have such a very Dear wife. Yes, honey, I was only kidding about you being sorry you married me. I know better, my Dear. I knew I'd get a rise out of you. Ha! Ha!

Goodnight my Dear and pleasant dreams.

[Thursday] September 14th

I don't know what's the matter with the mail from my parents? I didn't get any mail from home for the last three days. What's the matter! Is there anything the matter up home? If there's anything the matter please let me know.

Yesterday and last night I was just too busy to write and on top of that, I was pretty tired after the day. Please don't be angry with me, my dear.

In the afternoon we had three hours of marching and bivouac[28] and then at 4:00, we had to run the Obstacle Course, and boy that was something. That's tough and I mean tough. I was dead tired after I got through but I managed everything. Where the toughest part for me was crossing a body of water by walking your hands; that is, you grabbed a rope over your head and swung your body moving your arms at the same time. That is your arms supported your weight. I never thought I'd make it.

Then last night we had four hours of night operations. We were out on "reconnaissance" patrols. Got back by 11 PM and by 11:30 we had to be in bed. So, you see till I washed a little I couldn't have written a letter. You will forgive me won't you Dear?

---

[28] Term used for setting up a temporary encampment.

This morning we had two hours on how to put wounded men on litters and put them in an ambulance.

My Honey Bunch, if you or your Mother want to send me some food you can do so. I've run out of such things and a "midnight" snack comes in handy.

Honey, you'd probably like to come down with that Bowman girl, wouldn't you? Well, now let me tell you something. The way things look at the moment, I'll be here for the remaining of my Medical Basic, which is 8 more weeks. The last three we're on bivouac; that is, we're out camping somewhere and I wouldn't be able to see you during that time. Up to then, I'd probably be able to see you on weekends and night pass on Saturday. Some nights during the week when I have nothing to do in the evening you could come out to camp by bus and meet me at the Service Club and we could spend the night together up until 10 PM. Rooms, I hear, in Abilene run about $6 a week upwards. Now if you think it's worth coming, given those last three weeks of bivouac, why let me know immediately.

P.S. Yesterday, I received a steel mirror from Carpenter Steel Co. with my initials on it. It's very nice. It's worth quite a bit of money to buy it. I know for a fact that the steel used is very expensive stuff. I might send it home rather than keep it here.

[Friday] September 15th

At 5 PM I saw that I was on K.P. tomorrow again.

Gosh, but I'm lucky to have such a dear and true wife. I'm always looking at your picture. I can see your smile always before me.

This morning we had an exam in Materia Medica. I answered everything and I'm quite sure I had everything right. We also had an hour of Ward Medical Records and an hour on how to treat men for shock and an hour on the causes of disease (various types of bacteria).

This afternoon we had an hour on how to give blood and plasma transfusions and then we had a march with full field equipment. It was just four miles but it was a terrific pace. One almost had to run the whole way. I've never seen so many men fall out of a march. Our Company is setting a record for excellent marches.

Yes, I dream of you every night. It makes me sleep so well.

[Saturday] September 16th

My Dearest Sugar Plum,

As you know I was on K.P. today. That job is no different no matter what day, month, or year. Ha! Ha! I had plenty to eat too. I certainly will not lose any weight if they get me on K.P. very often. They had cocoa and gosh did I drink cocoa. Most of the meals we have coffee and when they have anything else, I really enjoy it and I get plenty of second, thirds and fourths.

I'm terribly sorry that your mail gets to you so late. You must tell your mailman to bring it to you more quickly; that your husband demands it and that he works for the government. Ha! Ha!

My dear, you tell me that you think I was in Abilene last Friday night. No honey, I was not. I couldn't go in if I'd want to. During your Basic Training, you can't leave the camp except for Saturday nights and on Sunday. That letter postmarked Abilene must have been neglected at Camp Barkeley so they stamped it when it hit Abilene-understand?

Thanks ever so much for getting me the paper. I saw in the paper that a Harold Kunkleman from Reading was killed in France in August sometime. I guess he's not related at all to your family, is he?

Yes, we'll have about three children. That's a nice number. I want at least one of each. How about it?

Did you kill those other roosters yet? You don't need an alarm clock when you have those things. They'll get you awake. I'm glad to hear that you are so fond of them. Are you feeding and taking care of them too? Ha! Ha!

[Sunday] September 17th

Hello Sweetest Apple Dumpling,

Now Dear, don't be disappointed when Wed. the 20th rolls around and there won't be any flowers coming. I had planned to wire you some flowers for your birthday but when I approached the Western Union place, I walked by a little Mexican shop that imported Mexican handicrafts and the like. It had a sign outside which stated it mailed goods anywhere in the U.S. So, I went in and I bought you something in there. Now they'll send it by mail and also insure it. However, it won't get to you probably until near the end of the week so don't think I forgot about your birthday. Never Dear, because on that day the sweetest woman was born that ever saw the light of day. I certainly wish we could celebrate it together but next year we'll make up for it. Maybe you won't think what I got you was very nice but they "sock" you so terribly much for things like that. You'll let me know as soon as you receive the gift, won't you?

Dear as you know I went to Abilene this afternoon. I went to the USO and they directed me to the Traveler's Aid Bureau. The girl who was there was very nice about it. They certainly try in every way to accommodate the soldier and his family. I asked how long ahead of time they'd have to know to get a room. She said that she'll get us one anytime you come. We must decide very shortly what to do.

All right dear, I'll give you the Yankees in the American League. I'll take the Browns for $.25. I guess you saw by today's paper that St. Louis is again in the lead by a 1/2 game. Should Detroit win out why the bet would be off. Is that right? We'll also have to bet on the World Series, too-how about it?

(birthday card with two roses on the front)-Happy Birthday to My Wife and Sweetheart

A birthday greeting from the heart,
For You and You Alone,
And it makes me mighty happy
Just to know that you're my own,
And all my heart belongs to you
For you're my SWEETHEART still,
It's You and You Alone I Love
And, dear I always will---Luke

[Monday] September 18th

My Sweetest Honey Child,

How do you like that for a salutation? Gee Whiz, I can't wait until evening comes so I can write to my honey darling. I'm so lucky to have a good and true wife as I have. There aren't any more like you.

Today I hit the jackpot as far as mail is concerned. I received five letters.

This afternoon we had an hour of Duties of Personnel at a Medical Regimental Detachment, an hour of Concealment and Camouflage and then we had another march with full equipment.

Ruth Dear, "gigged" means the same as given demerits. Yes, they certainly make you keep things just right. I have the best record for our barracks which contains 18 men. I have only one demerit from the first day. Another fellow didn't get any either until the other day, his shoes were about 1/4 of an inch out beyond the bed.

I don't believe the men know where they're going until they get on the train. I'd go to O.C.S. after my basic and then I'd have to wait until my name would come up. I'd be an officer in Med Corps as far as I know. However, that record I have with the carbine rifle might influence them to put me in the Inf.

Honey, the other night we were issued some of our winter clothing, among them our overcoat. Boy, do I look like a soldier in that thing. I also got my brass insignia representing the Medical Soldier. I'm really proud of that. We wear it on our blouse during the winter.

P.S. Honey, did you see what happened to the Yankees over the weekend? Those A's handed them some important defeats. Of course, the season still has two weeks to go. Anything can happen.

[Tuesday] September 19th

This morning we spent the whole four hours in the hospital and we're going to spend a lot more hours there. This morning we had two hours of lecture and two hours of actual practice at the things he lectured in. We were required to make a hospital bed with a patient in it. The patient is never uncovered and yet we put on all new sheets. Then we had to take temperatures on the patients orally (by mouth), axillary (under the arm), and rectally (through the rectum). We learned to take pulse and number of respiratory movements.

This afternoon we had two hours on how to treat bone fractures and two hours on how to transport Sick and Wounded over bodies of water.

Tomorrow morning, we have an 8-mile march with our usual full field equipment. Supposed to last 2 hours. We'll probably make it in less than that.

Honey, tomorrow's your birthday. Next year we hope it'll be different. Let me take this moment to congratulate my dear and wish her many, many more happy ones.

[Wednesday] September 20th

This letter I'm afraid will be quite short. From 7 to 11 PM we have another night problem. It involves another 7-mile march so we'll have 15 miles in all today. We also had a ceremonial parade practice this morning.

This afternoon we had two hours on Treatment of Casualties. We administered hypodermics to one another. An office was standing at my side when I shoved in the needle. He said it was a very good puncture. The fellow that gave it to me didn't jab me hard enough and pushed it in then. That hurts when a fellow does that.

Ruth Dear, you can come down anytime you please. Things are as indefinite as ever but I believe I'll be here for my full 17 weeks.

Glad you have a garage for the car. It helps a little, I guess.

[Thursday] September 21st

Gosh, you had very good news for me. So, you're coming down with the Bowman girl. Gosh, I can hardly wait to see you. Now tomorrow night I'll write a more detailed letter about everything. As far as I know, there are no changes in my status. If there is before Wed 27th I'll send you a telegram. Honey, I'll try to find out where you can phone to get word to me when you hit Abilene. As far as a room, don't worry about that. We'll get you one when you arrive.

Soon we'll see each other. Boy, will that be a happy day for both of us! Gee, I love you so much. Gosh, I can't say that often enough. The lights are going out. Sleep well, honey.

[Friday] September 22nd

In this letter, I'll start by explaining everything I know at the moment about coming down. Today when I read your letter you seem to be very nervous and jittery about coming down. Honey, darling, I don't know that I said you were unwise for coming down. Really, I believe I'll stay for my 17 weeks. However, I absolutely can't say that for sure. If you come at all, I figured that it would be nicer to come with somebody so I thought it would be nice to come with the Bowman girl. Now, honey, you do exactly what you want to do. It's perfectly all right either way. I'm of course very anxious to see you just as you are to see me.

Honey, I don't know the address of the Traveler's Aid. I know how to get there but don't know the street. Are you coming by Greyhound? I believe you are and the bus terminal is right at the Traveler's Aid Station. I'll try and get into Abilene this weekend sometime and find out again whether a room is available, but I'm sure there is. Now I don't think I'll be able to see you until Saturday night. I still haven't found out where you can phone to get in touch with me. On Saturday night I'll go into the Traveler's Aid and find out where you're at. If you let me know absolutely that you're coming next Saturday I'll try and reserve a room and then they can direct you right there.

I'm so glad you got such nice gifts from everyone. My Dear, did you get those things I had sent for your birthday? I hope you did because I certainly think they should be there by this time. Today we had an examination in Anatomy and Physiology. It was a scheduled two-hour exam. I got a 100%.

[Saturday] September 23rd

I received a letter from Mother's cousin. She said she saw you a few weeks ago and you told her that I like the Army. Did I ever tell you that? Ha! Ha! Ha!

Well, the Army isn't too bad either. If I wouldn't have such a dear wife and dear folks back home, I wouldn't mind it at all.

From 11 to 12 this morning we had our weekly inspection. The fourth platoon (the one I'm in) won 1st place in our Company for the second straight week. This morning I checked my clothing as I do every morning and found a button off on the sleeve of one of my shirts. I hadn't worn the shirt since last Sunday and every day up until today it was O.K. I have my suspicions that it was deliberately torn off by someone to get me gigged. They (some of them in the barracks) are getting envious of me because I haven't been gigged at all. I put the shirt in my locker and tonight I sewed on the button. Yes, I'm even beginning to sew now, believe it or not.

My Dearest, you seem quite undecided yet as to whether you're coming down next week or not. Well, Honey, that is entirely up to you. Believe me, I'm satisfied either way. Don't feel as though I'm hinting as to what you should do.

P.S. Yes, honey, I'm sure we'll have those children in the next seven years. Bet we'll have at least two boys.

[Sunday] September 24th

Well, honey, I've completed now eleven weeks in the Army.

If you come to Texas on Wednesday you probably won't even receive this letter but I'll write anyway until I know for sure that you're coming.

That was certainly thoughtful of your Father to pull your ears.[29] He didn't want to forget that. Did you let him pull them 23 times plus one to grow? Ha! Ha!

Honey, dearest, are you sure you still love me real, real much? Gosh, I hope so. Did you receive my gift yet?? You certainly should have by this time.

It looks as though neither of us will have picked the American League winner. I believe now that Detroit will come out on top. If you want the "Cards" I'll let you have them in the Series. I'll take the American League winner. Honey Bunch, always love me real, real much.

[Monday] September 25th

I wonder if you'll ever get this letter. Certainly, if you come to see your husband it will never get to you. Gosh, I can hardly wait to see what you'll do. Of course, I'm very anxious to see you. I can just imagine how I'll feel if you come but realize that there are so many uncertainties that I don't like to make up your mind for you.

This afternoon, we had two hours of Hand-to-Hand Combat, how to throw and kill your opponent with your hands. That's very interesting to learn.

On Wednesday we're going on a three-day problem-that is we're going out camping. We won't come back until 11 PM Friday. So, if you aren't on your way to Texas by this time you won't receive any letters for a few days. I see we'll have night problems every night out there so I can't see how I'll get anything written. Gee Whiz, for three nights I won't be able to write. I'm terribly sorry.

---

[29] There is an old tradition in several European countries to pull on your ear for every year of your birth with hopes of bringing good luck in the future.

Don't you worry dear if you think you'll hug me to pieces! What do you think I'll do to you? Yes, Dear, I can just imagine what I'll do when I see you!

No, my dear it certainly isn't cool down here. The days especially are hot.

Yes, Ruth darling, I'm afraid your Yankees are definitely out of the picture. It's between Detroit and St. Louis and now I believe the Tigers will win.

[Tuesday] September 26th

Gosh, I'm getting anxious to know what you're going to do tomorrow.

I guess you're wondering how I'm able to write at 11:00 in the morning. Well, I'm on Special Detail today only instead of being on K.P. there are two of us known as Room Orderlies. We sweep and mop the Company office and thoroughly clean the latrine. Well, we were finished by 10:30. We must remain in the office in case anything arises but I went down to my hut and got my writing paper. Nobody said a word about it so I guess it's all right.

Gosh, our packs will be quite heavy for the march to the bivouac area. I'm afraid we'll have to take two blankets along this time instead of only one because it might get rather cool in the evenings. I understand that the next three days while out on this problem we'll have to make lots of improvised splints and attach them to the legs and arms of other men. We have to imagine they are wounded in battle, give them first aid, and evacuate them to the nearest Medical Station.

Gosh, my dear, I can hardly wait until I know definitely whether you're coming down or not. I hope you tell me definitely in today's letter.

Honey Darling it's 1:15 PM and I've just cleaned up a bit around the place. I've decided to finish this letter now that I have a chance. I was rather disappointed this noon. I didn't get a letter from my Honey or Leesport.

[Ruth arrived in Abilene sometime after the 26th and stayed until around October 24th]

[Tuesday] October 24th

How's my Darling? Gee Whiz, I've been thinking about you so much this whole day wondering how your trip is coming. You should be somewhere around the Ohio State Line or probably in Ohio itself by this time. Have you met any nice people so far, I hope so? It makes your trip far less tiresome. How are your buses? Have you had all the good and new ones? Gosh, I wish I could make the trip with you. I like to travel so much when I'm with my Honey Bunch.

Well, I've put in two full days of Bivouac and I'm still in 100%. Again, I'm writing this by the light of the candle. It's amazing how many things one can do in the world. This kind of life makes a man rugged. Ha! Ha!

This morning we got up at 6:30. We had our breakfast (out of mess kits) and at 8 AM we had to establish a Collecting Station (a Medical Station in the 2nd Echelon of Medical Service to Wounded Troops). This afternoon we operated this Collecting Station. Wounded patients from the Battalion Aid Station were brought in for treatment. Every man had a particular job to do. Even when we eat, we assimilated battle conditions. We seek cover for everything we do. Planes are flying overhead constantly and will drop poison gas on us, at any time. We wear our gas masks all the time, even when we're in bed sleeping on the ground. Ha! Ha!

Well honey, I sure hope that you get home safely. I'll sure feel better at about 5 PM tomorrow. Gee Whiz, I wish you knew how much I love you and how wonderful I felt when I had the chance to see you. Always love me real, much. Love and Kisses Luke XXXX

[Wednesday] October 25th (on a postcard to Mr. and Mrs. Kunklemen- Ruth's parents)

Hello, my dear folks,

This afternoon I'm working in a Battalion Aid Station and I have a few minutes before my next casualty comes in so I thought I'd drop a few lines.

I guess Ruth will have a lot to tell you people about our experiences. I hope she gets to Reading in one piece. Ha! Ha!

This is my third day of bivouac. So far it hasn't been too bad. Hope to see you soon. Love Luke

[Thursday] October 26th

Gosh, I'm sure glad that your trip is over. I'm very much relieved to know that you're home. Are you resting well and taking things easy? Is everybody keeping you busy telling them about your trip? Did the bus at Harrisburg make good connections with the Reading Transportation Co. bus? You must write and tell me all about your trip home.

Honey Bun, I don't know what will happen about my writing. My candle stock is getting low and my writing paper won't last 17days. I'll try and get a hold of some more candles. If not, you'll know the reason for me not writing. I'll soon have to use cards instead of writing paper. Just remember everything is O.K. here at bivouac.

This morning my platoon again operated a Battalion Aid Station. This afternoon we operated a Clearing Station. This Station normally in battle is about 5-6 miles behind the front lines. I guess you don't understand this so well. I'll explain it when I get home if you want to know more about it.

Tonight, after chow, I had to sign more papers with regards to O.C.S. By gosh for the small chance we have of getting in they really do keep after you. The Commanding Officer wants to interview me out here on bivouac.

[Friday] October 29th

This is a Friday night. One more day and I'll have a full week in and I'm not regretting it a bit. This morning they woke us up at 2 AM. We had to roll our full field pack and fall out. We marched about 3-5 miles, had some "Demolitions" and "Incendiaries" thrown among us, came back at 7 AM. Everything is O.K. in Texas.

[Sunday] October 29th

Holy Smokes, you'll never know how good it made me feel to hear from you and to know that you got home safely. I'm sorry to hear that you had to stand for four hours. That must have been terrible.

Yesterday we had a field inspection. We had to display full field equipment in just the right manner in front of our "pup" tents.[30] The Commanding Officer told us that our "slit trenches" and "fox holes" were not deep enough. So, after a half-hour of Orientation, we had to start digging on our fortifications. I'm sure my slit trench is deep enough now. I can lay in it and have about 18-inch clearance.

Yesterday afternoon we had Mass Athletics all afternoon. I played softball.

This morning I ate breakfast and at 8:30 we had a Protestant church service. I, of course, went and the chaplain

---

[30] This was a two-man tent made up of two half pieces of water repellent, mildew resistant cotton and rayon duck with snaps along the ridge line. Each soldier carried a half plus poles, stakes and rope weighing about 5 lbs for each soldier. It should be pitched in 5 minutes and could also be used as a poncho or cover when it rained.

certainly had a fine service. The sermon was about the "Good Samaritan" who gave aid to the man who fell among thieves. He pointed out three philosophies of

life. 1) The one which the thieves held was "What is yours is mine and I'll get it even if I have to kill you". 2) The one which the priest and Levite had- "What is mine is mine and I'll keep it" and 3) the one which the Samaritan had- "What is mine is also yours". After the service, I shook his hand and told him how I thought that "Masons" taught such things too. He said yes indeed. He's also a 32nd Degree Mason. He was very glad to know that I was a Mason.[31]

Yes, Ruth, I wouldn't let that letter from the War Department scare you. It's just another routine for them to class a person "dead" after 12 months. His status really hasn't changed even then because they still haven't found a reason to pronounce him dead. Do you see what I mean? In the letter you got he was still termed as missing, wasn't he? I've borrowed this paper to write. I don't know where I'll get my next sheets. I'm afraid all I'll have soon is cards.

Don't forget to tell Sister to have those 8 A's for the Buick used before Nov. 8th. Either fill up the Buick and use the next for the Chevy or give them to Warren and allow us credit for later on. Just don't let them be wasted.

Yes, my Dear, I'm disappointed too about you being "sick". Something must be done. We absolutely want some children. Three boys are the best. Ha! Ha!

If I were you, I'd see the doctor again. Wait until I get home. I'll really "lay you out". Ha! Ha!

I saw in the Reading Times that Bruce was wounded for the third time. Gosh, that's tough.

---

[31] The Masons are a fraternal organization dating back to the 14th century centered on building character and strengthening communities.

Gee Whiz, I certainly wish that I could have made that trip home with you. I enjoy travel so much and observe everything. We'll really enjoy ourselves when the war is over. Nothing I can do is too good for my dear wife and our parents.

[Tuesday] October 31st

Honey Bunch, the last two days have probably been the toughest I've ever spent in the Army but I'm glad to say that I'm fine right now but about 8:30 this morning I was a bit weary.

My paper is scarce so I can only write this one sheet. At 4:30 PM they told us to roll our full field pack and fill our fox holes by chow time. After chow, we were taken to an adjoining field and put in definite formation. Then they told us that at 11:45 PM we'd be served some biscuits and coffee and that at 1 AM we'd ship out. We walked all night until 8:30 AM. Walked 25 miles to our new bivouac area. After we got here, we had to dig our foxholes and set up our pup tents.

Last night at 7:30 PM the Pocket Testament League[32] presented a short program out at Bivouac. They had a short film strip concerning the Bible. I saw part of it but rested about 10:30 to 11 PM.

[Wednesday] November 1st (11:20 PM)

Well Honey Bun, as you can see it's pretty late tonight but not knowing when I can write again, I'm going to send you a letter.

Tonight, we had a night program from 7 until 11 PM. We had about a six-mile march together with a map reading

---

[32] This was an Evangelical Ministry started in 1893 that provided the New Testament small enough to be carried in a shirt pocket. League Teams would visit military camps and hand them out.

program. We had to use our compasses to find our way back to camp. All in all, it wasn't too bad.

I was very fortunate again today; I received three letters from Pennsylvania. I forgot to tell you in yesterday's letter that we got paid-yes believe it or not they pay you right in bivouac. I received my usual amount of $21.21.

Well in a week from tomorrow we'll be heading back to Camp Barkeley and it can't come too soon for me. Ha! Ha!

Gee Honey, but you mustn't think that I'm too good for you. You're the best there is.

[Thursday] November 2nd

Guess what, I'm a litter bearer.[33] We're evacuating casualties from the Battalion Aid Station. It's hard work to haul patients on a litter but we have quite a bit of time between litter hauls. Tonight, we'll have to work until 11 PM so I'm glad to be able to get a few lines written now while the officers are being occupied. Tomorrow night I heard we work all night at a medical installation from 8 AM Friday until 8 AM Saturday and then carry on Saturday with our regular schedule.

Next Thursday morning we start back for Camp. Rumors have been spreading that a good portion of men from my company are going to "Cadre" School. Remember I had told you what that was. Holy Smokes, I hope I'm not one of those fellows but I can only wait to find out. I'm certainly anxious to find out just what will happen when we get back to Camp.

---

33 These soldiers carried the wounded as much as 4 miles over wooded and rocky terrain. Sometimes they setup relay teams during battle that would continue for hours. Shoulder straps were worn to insert the litter poles for easier transport.

I see my Honey is keeping track of the buses at her place. Well, that always interests me too.

Honey, the money you spend on my Christmas fund and other things for me I'll want to pay back, so please keep a record of all expenditures for my sake. Please.

[Friday] November 3rd

My Sweetest Dearest Apple Bun,

Today we're working in a Clearing Medical Station. This afternoon I'm assigned here to the "Shock Section". We must as a very first treatment give plasma.[34] They'll make a Medical man out of me yet. Ha! Ha!

The nights which follow the problems, I can sleep on that hard ground as though it were an innerspring mattress. Ha! Ha!

[Saturday] November 4th

From eight to ten we had an inspection. However, at 7:30 they gave the call that I was supposed to be interviewed by the Battalion O.C.S. Board, which includes my Company Commander, Battalion Commander, and one other officer. Well, I appeared at the designated Command Post at the designated time, had to wait until 10 AM before I was told to come in. It only lasted about 15 minutes, but boy did they fire the questions at me. Things that didn't even have anything to do with MAC or even my training. One question they asked me I had no idea what the answer was so I immediately said "I don't know, Sir". They seemed pleased that I answered

---

[34] Plasma is a component of blood made up of mostly water. It could be dried, stored for some time and reconstituted when needed. Since it doesn't contain red blood cells no cross match was needed. It helped with volume and electrolyte loss and maintaining blood pressure but didn't provide the red cells needed for oxygen transport.

immediately rather than stall around. Afterward, I found out that is what they like-to answer quickly and directly even if you don't know the answer. One must appear before two more boards the way I understand the matter. It seems so useless, however, since they pick so few men anyway.

[Sunday] November 5th

Today is another very welcome Sunday. It's nice to have a day completely to oneself every once in a while. All you have to do is rest, go to religious services, write letters and eat and boy, I certainly don't miss that last thing!

It seems that on Sundays we have the best meals for the whole week. This morning we had pancakes (I had four), oatmeal, stewed prunes, stewed apples, bread and butter, and milk. This noon we had ham, sweet potatoes in molasses, peas and lima beans, salad, Jell-o, and lemonade. It was all very good yet some complained it wasn't enough. Well, I had plenty. I doubt if you could satisfy some people no matter what or how much you'd feed them.

This morning we had church services. Well, I was there at 8:30 but there were very few men there, in fact, I was the only one from my Company. One of the officers of the Battalion saw there were so few that he asked us to go back to our Company areas and try and muster up some more men. Just as I got to my area the 1st Sgt. was calling the Company together and this same officer was telling him to announce the services. He did so and asked all those who wanted to go to service to step out. I was the only one who stepped out. He gave the company a lecture for not more wanting to go to church. Finally, about 10 more men stepped out and we went to service.

Yesterday I had another new experience which I never thought I'd have especially if I was in this Country. On Friday night before we were dismissed at chow the announcement was made that tomorrow, we'd cook our meals. Boy oh boy, was that something. For breakfast, we had to boil our eggs and for dinner and supper, we had to cook our meat and potatoes. Well, I didn't do bad. We built a fire and we fixed things up rather well. The meat was rather rare but that didn't matter.

[Monday] November 6th

Gee whiz, I feel I'd better write quickly as I possibly can for fear of not being able to later on. Today I've been rather fortunate. I've been picked as a "casualty". I've been placed out beyond our Medical Installation in the line of Battle. I was given a tag that indicates what's the matter with me. I've received, according to the tag, extensive wounds of the shoulder. I'm now awaiting medical treatment by the company aid man and then further evacuation through the Medical Installations. Once my arm and shoulder are dressed, I'm afraid I won't be able to write.

Honey, you've been asking my opinion on buying Christmas cards as to what and how you wanted them printed. It doesn't matter one bit to me as to whether I'll be a "Pvt." by Christmas. Of course, maybe you'd prefer Luke and Ruth or Mr. and Mrs. Even if I would get a P.F.C. or anything else I wouldn't mind having "Pvt." on the card. Why not ask your parents and my parents for advice.

Honey Bunch, I'm sorry to hear that you're not anxious for Christmas. Even if Howard and I are not able to be there you must just remember that wherever we are we're enjoying the happy times that exist in our own families and we certainly wouldn't feel good if we knew that you weren't enjoying yourselves. Remember, I'm happy only if you're smiling. I'm smiling even if I'm not beside you in person, I am in mind and spirit. Remember that.

Honey, don't worry about gifts. We have plenty of money in the bank. Use it to buy gifts because that's the way I want it. Just believe that I'm right with you and that Howard is too.

[Tuesday] November 7th

Gee whiz, my Dear, things have happened so fast the last 24 hours that I'm still in a daze.

Let me start at the minute they woke me up this morning at 6:30. At that time while I was still asleep, I heard the Sgt. yell- all O.C.S. men be prepared to go into camp at 7:15. Gee Whiz, we had to prepare our strip packs and eat and be ready to leave at 7:15. Well, they brought us in by truck. We had to shave and get "spruced" up by 9:30 to go before the Regimental O.C.S. Board. I was kept stepping. I felt like a new man to be able to take a good hot shower and get in my class A. uniform.

At 9:30 we went up to the Board. I was called in third and they really give you a workout. They fired questions at you at a terrific pace. I felt much more at ease than I did at the Battalion interview. They even asked me the Generals of our Armies as well as who were the heads of the cabinet posts. They couldn't catch me at such questions. I have no idea how I made out. I must go before one more board yet before I'm finished. They certainly make you go through a lot of interviews just to tell you that you were rejected. Ha! Ha!

The clerk in the office gave some of us detail work in the afternoon. I was varnishing some tables all afternoon. At 4:30 the clerk came back and told me I'd go back to the Bivouac Area at 7:30 tonight. Well, at 6:00 those plans were changed and I was put on guard duty from midnight until 2 AM. As far as I'm concerned, I'd rather varnish tables and walk guard duty, and be able to sleep on a mattress rather than sleep on the hard ground. According to the schedule, we'll march in on Thursday morning so they'll surely take me out by tomorrow night so that I can walk in the following morning. This evening I got a haircut at the PX. Gosh, I needed a haircut too.

Gosh, the mail has failed to catch up with me for the last two days. I didn't receive a bit of mail yesterday or today.

Honey Bun, you've been asking me what I want for Christmas. Dearest, you know I have no preference at all. I don't know what I need. I have everything that any man could ask for. I think you shouldn't bother with me at all. Ha! Ha!

[Thursday] November 9th

Yesterday morning and early afternoon I again varnished tables. At 3 PM I went out to the Bivouac Area. We had to roll our full field packs and police our area thoroughly. Gosh, it got cold last night too, and guess what, we had to sleep on the ground since our tents were rolled in our packs. At 3:45 we got up and ate breakfast and started marching in at 4:45. A couple of us built a fire to keep warm during the night. I'm glad I have a little "speck" to help keep warm. Ha! Ha! Ha!

We hit camp at 9:40 AM. It was a pretty long march- about 15 miles. When we got to our area the whole Camp Barkeley band was there to greet us and the Commanding Officer of our whole Regiment was standing in review as we passed. It was an honor paid to our Battalion by Colonel Darby.

As soon as we arrived at our area the 1st Sgt. read off a list of 8 men who were supposed to appear before the head O.C.S. Board. It's the last board that interviews the men and lo and behold my name was one of those 8 men. I appeared before the Board at 2 PM. There were Colonels and Majors on the Board. I felt nervous when I went in but once I did get in, they seemed very "common" and I was quite calm. I was very well pleased with the interview. They even asked me capitols of States and they couldn't catch me on a single one. They asked me so many different kinds of questions. I don't know now what will happen.

Well, my Dear, the election is over and I'm certainly well pleased. Roosevelt[35] won in a landslide. Even I didn't think he'd win by the majority he did. Yes, the people know he's doing a great job. I even see it more since I'm in the Army. I'd have hated to see a new man get in. I'm very glad to hear you voted the straight Democratic Ticket. As a rule, I don't do that either but this time I also voted the Democratic Ticket straight because they all were fairly good men. Also, glad to hear that your Aunt Sally and Aunt Ruth were on the right side of the fence.

[Friday] November 10th

This morning we had two hours of Orientation, an hour on the Article of War, and an hour on Military Courtesy.

That was mighty nice of your Father to go around by way of "Wagner's" to get that ice cream and also to get gas in the Buick. According to Sister, the Buick's tank is full and there are 25 gal. worth of gas coupons that Stoudt has for our later use. Gosh, I don't even believe that I can use all that when I get home. Ha! Ha!

Honey Bunch, you must use your influence in making a "good girl" out of your manager. It's just too bad that a

---

[35] Franklin D. Roosevelt served as President from 1933 until his death in 1945. Stricken with polio in 1921 he suffered permanent paralysis from the waist down allowing him only to stand or walk short distance wearing iron braces on his hips and legs.

married woman must carry on like that especially when her husband is risking his life every minute of the day.

Well, they are starting to ship some men out of our Company already. They've been assigned. I can hardly wait to see what will happen.

Honey, you must take care of your cold. Gee Whiz, I'm worried about you. You had that cold when you were down here and still have it.

[Sunday] November 12th

Well, here I am spending this Sunday at Camp Barkeley and it's much nicer writing in a bed than it is on the ground.

Yesterday I was on K.P. and at 6:45 a soldier came up to the kitchen and asked for me. I went to the door and guess what- there was Victor Mogel. He's a brother of Stanley, you know his twin brother. They're my Mother's cousins. Gosh, it was good to see him. He's in the 60th Medical Battalion and was on bivouac the last three weeks also. He's waiting to be assigned. We talked and talked and talked and it was 9:30 PM when he left. I was sorry that I didn't get a chance to write my Honey Darling. I only hope she'll forgive me.

This morning I went to church. It was a memorial service for all the men who have died in the war. The chapel was rather full too. I'll forgive you and your Father for not going last Sunday especially if you had company and your Father didn't feel well. I hope, however, that you went today.

Dearest, why in the world don't you go to a doctor for your cold? You absolutely must go or your hubby is going to whip you when he sees you again. Ha! Ha! All kidding aside please get your cold looked after.

Darling, you worry about that car of ours too much. You mustn't think that I'll "bawl" you out for leaving the brake on.

[Monday] November 13th

Gee Whiz, I'm so anxious to know what will happen to me. Everybody's wondering. I have no idea whatsoever. I've heard all sorts of rumors and I don't believe any of them.

How are your parents? I certainly hope they're all right. I can't wait to taste some of your mother's good cooking and her good custard and cakes. Yum! Yum!

I haven't heard from O.C.S. for the last couple of days. I understand they definitely tell you if you're turned down or rejected. Yes, the physical exam will be difficult. I'm told that they might reject me even if I would be accepted otherwise.

Yes, Honey, $31.54 was good money. I'm quite sure those shoes you bought were very pretty. Gosh, my dear always dresses so nicely and looks so beautiful.

Sorry to hear about Uncle Allen. Yes, being gassed often brings on complications later on in life. I hope he's better by this time. Glad your cold is somewhat improved. That makes me feel better.

[Tuesday] November 14th

Today is another beautiful day in Texas. It's amazing how warm it can be in the middle of November when it's just about freezing at home.

I was somewhat disappointed this noon when the mailman failed to have a letter from Pennsylvania for me. Of course, we have another mail call this evening and I hope there's some mail there for "Pvt. Snyder".

I was called out twice for detail work. We cleaned the windows and scrubbed the walls of the latrine until you could see yourself in the wood. Ha! Ha! Gosh, that place was never so clean. In the meantime, they have very little for us to do. Our classes are all finished and all there is to be done is detail work of some sort.

Gosh, there's so little I can write about that I guess I'll close for now.

[Wednesday] November 15th

Gosh, it feels like winter today. The skies are overcast and if I'd be in Penna. I'd say that it would snow any minute.

Today we're doing very little again. This is getting quite monotonous. Yesterday afternoon we had to clean up under the barracks. There were a lot of beer bottles and pop bottles that were thrown under. This morning and this noon again certain men were called out for detail work.

Well, this morning at 7 AM and this afternoon at 1:30 there were two more groups of men shipped out. Everyone here is just waiting.

Honey, were there any Armistice Day celebrations around Reading? Did business go on as usual? Here in Abilene, I understand they had quite a big parade of all men who were overseas.

Honey Dear, I'm shocked at the way you talked in your letters. I'm surprised at my wife. Honey, you should be ashamed!! Ha! Ha! Just what did you mean in your Saturday letter when you said "we'd be able to have a "----" every night". I can't in the world imagine what you meant except having a "----" every night and if that is what you meant, I'm surprised by my wife. Then in Sunday's letter, she wrote about giving me the "works" even if she was sick. Boy My Honey seems to mean business!! Well, if she wants it that bad, she's really going to get it, so much she won't be able to take any more. Remember how "it" felt down there some weekends. Ha! Ha!

Darling, how is your cold? Believe me, my dear, I wish you'd get some medicine for that cough. That is a terrible strain on a person to have to be coughing continually.

[Thursday] November 16th

Gosh, today is awful dreary. It's cold and chilly. I believe up in Pennsylvania we'd have had snow instead of rain.

Gosh, I never dreamed that the Army would ever allow you so much free time. I presume they figure they've worked us pretty hard the last seventeen weeks and they want to give us a rest before our next assignment. I wish they'd soon make up their minds.

I haven't heard a thing yet from O.C.S. Yesterday some of the fellows received their notice from the O.C.S. board that they were rejected and the reason why. Nobody was accepted yet so I guess you must just wait and see what happens.

Last evening "Ed" asked me if I'd play some ping pong with him. Since I had already written home, I told him I would. Gosh, I hadn't played that game for some time. I beat him about 5 straight games and then another fellow challenged me after watching us play. I also beat him a game then he quit.

Golly, my Dear, I don't know what to say about getting our furniture. How much do we still owe on it? What would you rather do in the matter? Dear, as far as drawing the money from the bank that's perfectly all right. Sooner or later, we'll have to pay it anyway. I don't think you should use the Christmas Club money. That you use for other things. Gosh, it'll be rather hard for me to get all my Christmas shopping done.

I'm so glad your cold is better. Now keep taking your medicine faithfully.

[Friday] November 17th

Again, I hardly know what to write. I haven't done a thing so far today. We all are restricted to our barracks; I presume to be sure we're around if and when our names are called for shipment. I've been reading "Look Magazine"[36] this morning and getting plenty of rest. Even civilian life isn't as easy as this. Ha! Ha!

Honey, you mustn't keep that Chevy spotlessly clean. Heavens, it never was that way when I was home.

Dearest, I can hardly believe that you and Sister are becoming so very good at that game of Rook. My, the women won't let you play with them anymore. Ha! Ha! Gosh, I can hardly believe that Sister is beginning to like Rook. I'm glad though because now you have a foursome.

So, the big pussy was hit again? I can't see that she can be so lucky. Wasn't she hit a few times before?? Is she getting better?? How are Judy and the other pussy getting along?

I'm sorry about your Father's Rheumatism. He isn't getting enough rest. Really, he's working too hard. How is your Mother? Is she all right? I hope-and your grandparents-are they okay? I hope the election hasn't disappointed them too much. How come your Aunt Ruth and Aunt Sally were for Roosevelt amid all those Republicans??

[Luke left Camp Barkeley for furlough home on November 18th until November 29th]

---

[36] This magazine was published from 1937 to 1971 emphasizing photographs. It cost 10 cents an issue and $2.50 for a yearly subscription in 1944. The March 1945 cover was Rita Hayworth.

Reassigned to Camp Swift-10th Mountain Division

[Thursday] November 30th

Since you insist on having me write on the train you must put up with poor penmanship. The train rocks too much to have me write plainly. We're traveling between Columbus, Ohio, and Dayton, Ohio at this moment. We left Columbus at 9:15 and are due in Dayton at 10:40. We left Harrisburg last night at 11:40- yes thirty minutes late, but by the time we reached Pittsburg we were only 5 minutes late and now we're exactly on time, so there is no fear that we'll miss that 6:00 train out of St. Louis.

Gee Whiz, but I love my wife so very much. Gosh, she was so very good to me while I was home. I certainly can easily understand why everyone likes you, My Dear. How did you get home last night? From what I've seen you drive very well. You must be sure and tell me all about it when you get my address.

Guess what, it's been snowing since about 1:30 this morning and right now it's really coming down. Everything is covered with snow and it's starting to pile up. I wonder if it's snowing in Berks right now? I hope my Honey enjoyed herself during the last week or so. I had such a nice time.

Right now, the train has hit Dayton and I'm able to write a bit. By gosh, Uncle Sam is still drafting men. Right outside our window, there are about two dozen fellows that are just being drafted into the service waiting to board the train for an induction center. So, the way things look there is still a war on. Ha! Ha! Ha! If they only knew what they're getting into?

Just before I started this letter, I ate a tangerine. That's all we had so far. You don't have to worry about me not having enough to eat. Ed has a package full of sandwiches and cookies and Zerby too has a lot of food. I'm sure we won't lose any weight on the train.

Honey Bunch I owe you so much money I'll be paying you back the rest of my life. Gee, you're buying these Christmas gifts now yet together with that $50.00 you gave me for my trip home. Yes, it was mighty good to be home. I certainly enjoyed every minute of it. I'm sorry we didn't get time for a "----" before I left but I don't think you wanted it very badly. Ha! Ha! By Gosh, something should develop from all those "rendezvous" we had together. Ha! Ha!

[Saturday] December 2nd

As you probably guess I'm writing this at Camp Swift.[37] I can't tell you much about the camp thus far because I haven't seen too much of it. Right now, we've laid out all our equipment and are waiting for someone to inspect it. In the meantime, there doesn't seem to be anything to do so I'm starting a letter.

We arrived at Austin, Texas at 5:30 PM, yes only 10 minutes late. Our train came into St. Louis at 5:20 PM. Yes, it ran late through Indiana and Illinois but we still had plenty of time to get the 6 PM train for Ft. Worth. It didn't leave St. Louis until 6:45 PM and we hit Ft. Worth on time (11:40 AM yesterday) and Austin at 5:30 PM. We really had some long drive. If only my Honey Bun was with me, we'd have enjoyed the trip quite a bit, wouldn't we? Ed, Zerby, and I were together most of the trip and we finished up all our "lunches" by about 2 PM.

After getting to Austin, we ate dinner and got a bus for Camp Swift. First, we picked up our barracks bags at the

---

[37] This Camp began as a training base in 1942, named after Major General Eben Swift. The 10th Mountain Division trained here in 1944. It is currently owned by the Texas Army National Guard.

station. They were shipped you know from Camp Barkeley. That really was a job dragging those bags around. Both of them weigh about 110lbs.

After we hit the Camp a truck took us to the 10th Division Headquarters. From there (there were eight of us that came here at that particular time) we were told where to go. I was sent to the 85th Unit along with Ed, as well as two other men. We were given two blankets and a bunk until morning.

It seems as though we're attached to an Inf. Division in the Regimental Aid Group. What we'll be doing I have no idea. The rumors are flying right and left.

Hon, now don't get any wild ideas because of the APO number. We are attached to a Mountain Inf. Group but we don't know when we're shipping out. I was told we're getting about two months of mountain climbing. Isn't that something? Ha! Ha!

[Sunday] December 3rd

I guess you are just going home from church about now or you are home by this time. Last Sunday I was with my Dear and I can just imagine where she was sitting and the like. They certainly leave you to do anything on a Sunday. You don't have to get up for breakfast and there is no roll call. As a result, I slept until 9:30 and then I got up, found the nearest chapel, and went to services. The chaplain is a quiet young man and he has a foreign accent of some kind but he's a very forceful and excellent minister. The theme of his sermon was "The Meaning of Religion".

As you can see by my address, I'm attached to the 85th Mountain Infantry. Well, that's what William was in. I say was because I looked him up after church this morning and found out he was transferred to the 86th Infantry last Saturday and the whole 86th Regiment shipped out of Camp Swift on Monday.

This afternoon Ed and I walked across camp to where some of the other men are stationed that came here from Camp Barkeley. We've eaten fine meals here since we arrived and Ed and I have eaten in four different mess halls. Everywhere you look there's a mess hall and whenever we hear a cook yell "chow is ready" we run. We're sampling the cooking of all the cooks. Ha! Ha! Ha!

Honey Darling, reports have it that I won't be at Camp Swift very long. The 1st Sgt. told me personally yesterday that the 85th Regimental Commander traveled to Camp Barkeley personally and picked out 31 men that had to meet certain qualifications for this 85th Inf. for the Medical Detachment. All 31 of us have College experience.

[Monday] December 4th

Gosh, my Dear, I hope you won't be angry at me for what I forgot to write earlier. Please, forgive me. Late Saturday afternoon the mail clerk gave us our mail that had been forwarded from Barkeley. Gosh, I received a lot of letters and I enjoyed reading every one of them so very much. I received four from you, really five since the one had two letters in it. It seems rather funny to read those letters now of how you're expecting me home and knowing that I was home in the meantime. Gosh, I had such a grand and glorious time. Yes, I even wore out my wife one night. Ha! Ha! It was so "tight" I couldn't get in. Ha! Ha! Ha! You'd better keep it "open" so I can get in anytime I come home. Ha! Ha!

Gosh, Honey, I forgot something else. On Saturday afternoon we got another shot. It was a typhoid injection. We're going to get two more within a very short time.

We still haven't been assigned to our permanent barracks as yet. This morning we've been sweeping out this temporary Headquarters and mopped it and piled all the mattresses in one corner. I've been told that our outfit has been put on alert. That means we're liable to ship out of here any day. Where to, I really don't know? If a man is absent from his post one minute without leave, he is considered a deserter which is punishable by death. If a group is alerted and a man is absent without leave, he is just considered AWOL which is, of course, not as serious an offense as being a deserter.

Now listen to me, my Dear, if by chance I should ever go overseas I think I'd increase my bond allotments and take out $18.75 a month and get a $25 bond. You see I'd receive $60 a month instead of $50 and they say you don't need much money over there.

Honey, what do you want for Christmas? Gee Whiz, the last few days I've been trying to think what you'd like to have. I must try and visit Austin and do some Christmas shopping. Gosh, being in the Army leaves one at a disadvantage in things such as that. If you have something in mind please let me know.

[Tuesday] December 5th

Yesterday afternoon, 31 men that are attached to the 85th Inf. were assigned to our respective Battalions. I was assigned to the 3rd Battalion. Unfortunately, Ed and I are separated. Ed has been asking everyone possible to have us transferred to the other one's outfit.

Yesterday afternoon the Captain of our outfit who is, I believe, our Regimental Surgeon gave us a short interview. This morning the 1st Sgt. called each one of us up to his bunk and interviewed us. He told us that the 3rd Battalion is by far the best battalion of the whole Regiment and he is very glad to have all the new men that were assigned.

[Wednesday] December 6th

This morning it was quite cloudy and gee- for Texas it's getting pretty cold. I got out the tops of my heavy underwear. Yesterday afternoon after I had written you, we had to install some more beds in our barracks.

I didn't see Ed at all yesterday until "Retreat". All the Medics stand Retreat at the same place and naturally at the same time. He managed to see me and we ate together. He's so disgusted that we're not together. We walked down to the nearest Service Club which is about 2-3 miles.

As you know we're attached to the 85th Mountain Infantry which is part of the 10th Mountain Division.[38] This Infantry is known without a doubt as one if not the best regiment of its kind in the U.S. Army, if not in the world. This infantry, and also some Medics who were attached to them before this time, had trained at Camp Hale, Colorado, and were known as the "ski" troops. Well Honey Bunch, in the next two months we're going to get training in the mountains. We are going to learn to ski, to live in extremely cold weather, to climb mountains and the like. We Medics will have to render medical aid to these infantry troops if and when they go into combat. Right now, some of us Medics know exactly what we'll do. Either we're "Company Aid Men" who work right on the front line giving First Aid or

---

[38] Designated as a mountain warfare unit it was originally the 10th Light Division (Alpine) located at Camp Hale, Colorado. The unit moved to Camp Swift in 1944 and was renamed and fought in the mountains of Italy in 1945. The unit was deactivated after the war but was permanently reactivated in 1985. Since then, they have been instrumental in several operations most recently in Iraq and Afghanistan.

"Evaluation Specialist", who must evacuate the casualties to the rear. There are 38 Medical Soldiers attached to one Infantry Battalion. There are 12 Company Aid Men, 18 Evacuation Specialists, and 8 men in the Battalion Aid Station. There were already 24 Medics attached to this Battalion and 14 of us new fellows.

[Thursday] December 7th

This morning we had about 1 1/2 hours of Physical Conditioning and Close Order Drill. Then we were called into one of the Day Rooms for a lecture. We were told what jobs we'd start in at and guess what I got into-what is normally termed a litter bearer. However, this outfit has termed them, evacuation specialists. One of the Non-Commissioned Officers definitely wanted me on his team. He asked for me personally. It certainly didn't appeal too much to me. There are six men in a team, normally four but the Mountain Evacuation requires six. Well, I'm second in command of our team. It's been the first real job I've had in the Army.

Tomorrow the whole Infantry Regiment will be given several shots and I'm supposed to help with these injections. It'll be all day and probably night as well. This afternoon I'm to report to the Dispensary to get my instructions.

Honey, I just saw that I didn't get any mail yet from home. By tomorrow I feel as though I should have a few letters-how about it?

Gosh, it's 1 PM right now. All the other Medics fell out for the afternoon except myself and the other Non-Commissioned officers who are going down to the Dispensary at 2 PM. I feel sort of out of place with all these older Army men. I hope I'll be able to do my job well.

[Friday] December 8th

Gosh, was I glad this noon when I received your letter. Honey, believe me, I almost cried for joy. I was so happy I read it at least 4 times, every word on every page, so you can see how anxious I was to hear from you. I just got the letter at 12:45 and at that time we were supposed to start giving injections. Well, I asked another fellow to do injections for me until I read your letter. I gave injections for typhus, typhoid, and the like with old Army men who were Corporals, Sergeants, and even higher. We injected about 500 to 800 men. About the first 10 I did I was rather nervous but after that, it wasn't so bad. You see you must change needles after each injection. Everything must be perfectly sterile. A fellow feels more like himself when he's able to do a job like that.

Here at Camp Swift, there is a G.I. laundry that does washing for the soldiers. You can deposit 25 pieces of clothing a week for $1.50 a month.

Gosh, I was certainly shocked to hear about Eugene. Gee, one never knows what to expect in war. I hope and pray that he's alright. That submarine "business" is a rather dangerous job, no question about it.

Gee Whiz, I'm worried so much about Grandma. How is she anyway?? How did she fall??? Please Honey Bunch tell me everything about how things are at home.

[Saturday] December 9th

Honey, do you have another boyfriend?? Ha! Ha! I believe it since I didn't get a letter from you this noon. The one you wrote on Wed. night I should have received today, but I didn't. I guess you must have gone out with the boyfriend. By the way, didn't you and Sister go into the Crystal Bar last Wednesday night after leaving the Outer

Street Station? You two said you were going in to see your two men friends. Aren't you two ashamed for doing such things? Ha! Ha! Ha!

I'm so interested that all of you have a happy Christmas. Honestly, that would make me feel so good to know that everyone back home is having Christmas just like before. If you want me happy that's what you'll have to do.

Mother also said that George was killed in action. Heavens, he left the same time that Earl left. Sister wrote in her letter that you and she had a conference in her room on Wednesday night trying to see what I was going to do. Well, I'm not even sure but I'm quite sure I'll render 1st Evacuation Medical Service. Eventually, I'll command all the litters or evacuation squads when and if we ever get into combat.

[second letter Saturday] December 9th

This is my second letter today and it'll be a very short one for the U.S.O is ready to close and I must get out. I'm writing this from the U.S.O. in Austin. Ed and I came to town to do a little shopping and believe it or not I bought something and already sent it. Now listen to this very carefully. You're getting a package sent to you from me. I don't want that opened until Christmas Day. Promise me that you will, won't you? You may not open it until Christmas Day. Understand? Gosh, I'm so happy to be able to buy my Honey a gift.

[Sunday] December 10th

Hello, my Sweetness! Boy was I lucky today. I received four letters again. Gosh, I could hardly wait until dinner time to receive my mail. Yes, I got two from my honey, the ones you wrote last Wednesday and Thursday.

Last evening, Ed and I came into town, and gosh do you have a time getting into Austin. By God, a fellow must be crazy to wait so long but we waited. We were in line from 5:30 until 7:20, before we got on a bus. Well, it took us 1 hour to get in! We got there at 8:20. I did some shopping, got a bite to eat, wrote a letter home at the U.S.O. and came back to Camp. It was after midnight when the bus got back to Camp Swift.

This morning I didn't get up for breakfast. I stayed in bed until 9:30 and then got up and went to church. Boy, it got real, real cold during the night. The wind is blowing at a terrific gale. Yes, it can get pretty cold in Texas.

Honey, please do not worry about me. I'm perfectly all right. You mustn't worry about me going overseas. I'll be careful and there's nothing to worry about.

You asked about mules???[39] All the mules have been shipped out before we came. They had a few thousand of them and the way I understand it we won't see the mules till about March. Where we'll see them, I don't know.

So, you refused a piece of chocolate cake! Yes, that certainly is willpower. I'm quite sure I wouldn't have that much willpower. But you don't have to lose weight, Honey, you're not too heavy in the least. Believe me. You tell Sister that she's all wrong in having you worry about the nurses! Heavens, I haven't even seen a nurse and I'm not at all interested because I have absolutely the Dearest and Best woman in the whole world, my Darling Wife.

Dearest, I know my O.C.S. application is still on file but the 10th Division will not release me at this time. They claim you're too vital a part of this organization.

---

[39] Mules were shipped overseas to be used as transport in rugged terrain. "Mule Skinners" were soldiers trained in the use and care of the animal. They were useful in the mountains of Italy.

[Monday] December 11th

I received a Christmas card today from the Service Mothers and Wives Committee of Leesport. Say I thought George had been killed in action. Evidently, Mother must have made an error in her letter. I see he was just missing. Isn't that funny? He was declared missing exactly a year to the day that he was inducted.

By Gosh, you can't imagine how cold it can get here in Texas. This morning while out marching my hands got terrifically cold. When I got back to the barracks, I took my gloves along. It's a beautiful day, however. I don't believe there's a cloud in the sky.

Honey, you'll soon be skin and bone if you continue to lose so much weight. Now please don't carry that diet too far. Be sure you get proper nourishment.

[Tuesday] December 12th

This morning we had an hour of Close Order Drill and Physical Conditioning. They are giving us plenty of calisthenics lately. We had an hour and 1/2 of lectures on Map Reading and an hour of Physiology. These lectures we're getting are almost solely a repetition or review of that same subject we had at Barkeley. It seems as though they're just marking time until leaving Camp Swift in about one week. You should hear the rumors fly as to where we're going. This could include training in the Rockies, in the mountains of Canada, or the mountains of Scotland, Southern France, or Central Italy. You hear reports that have us going to all five places. China was another rumor but I doubt that. I'm quite sure if we go overseas it will be to the European Theater.

Honey Bunch, you asked me about how much money to give the pastor and also in the current expense envelope. Honey, I'm afraid you'll run too short if you don't get money from the bank or use your allotment check. Put $100 in the current expense envelope and either $2.00 or $3.00 in the pastor's portion of the other envelope.

[Wednesday] December 13th

Today's routine was similar to the past few days. This afternoon there were further lectures and film strips. All of them had to do with the Censorship of Mail. It was all very dull as I had practically everything at Barkeley. It's amazing though how much these older men in the service do not know. Officers ask various questions in class. All of it should be known and by God, some of these old Army men who should know it look bewildered when they are called upon. We buck privates make them look silly. Ha! Ha!

Dearest, you asked me many times about what to get your Father. Have you given up on the idea of seat covers? Those at Firestone were very nice but I realize they were rather expensive. Does he need any kind of clothing-slippers or the like? Clothing is just about the only other thing I can think of.

Did you receive that box I sent home? It should just about be home by this time. It's insured. Does the mailman always make you sign for insured parcels?? I'm very interested in knowing that you received the parcel and Dear you won't open it will you?? You'll have less than two weeks to wait. My Gosh, I never thought Christmas was so close. We'll have a lot to make up for when this war is over. Everybody is going to be so happy. We're going to enjoy life every minute. We'll make everyone happy around us too, won't we, my Dear??

[Thursday] December 14th

How's my Dearest Apple Pie tonight? Gosh, I always feel good when I'm able to write to my Dear Wife. It's always such a nice way to finish a day. I always can dream of such nice thoughts.

Today was really a messed-up day if I can call it such. This morning we turned in our pack covers, pistol belt, and canteen cover and got all new stuff. The rest of the morning we were put on various detail work. I was cleaning up leaves around the barracks. This afternoon I turned in practically all my clothing and equipment and received new equipment. Things are starting to boom around here. I seem to have trouble finding a raincoat that fits me. The one I've been having was much too small. Well, I asked for a larger size. I came back to the barracks, tried it on. and my gosh, it was way too big so I go back, and finally, I got one that fits fairly well. After we were issued our new clothing, we were told that every piece of equipment had to be marked with your last initial and last four numbers of your serial number.

Honey, I wish you wouldn't send me any more gifts or anything. If we go overseas, I wouldn't feel like taking those things with me unless they're small. You see we are only allowed to have 7 lbs. of things that are not GI. I'm quite sure that I have a bit more than 7 lbs. now and I'll have to send some home.

I forgot to mention it. I hit the jackpot as far as packages go. I received three packages, mind you, one from Mother which contained my clean shorts, undershirts, and socks, as well as delicious cake, candy, and pretzels; a box from Pomeroy's[40] which contained pretzels, and a box from the Soldiers Wives and Mothers Committee of Leesport. By gosh, with all this food, it will be my fault if I starve. Ha! Ha! Ha!

---

[40] This was a department store founded in 1876, located in downtown Reading, Pa. It expanded to Harrisburg, Pottsville and Wilkes-Barre. The final closing came in 1990.

As a rule, Honey Bunch, my evenings are "free". I don't believe there is a bed check here. I have never heard anything to that effect. The lights in the barracks, however, must be out by 10 PM. We get up at 5:45 and have "reveille" at 6:15 and breakfast at 6:30.

Say, the way the papers talk, you must have had quite a bit of snow in Pennsylvania. I saw that in parts of West Virginia they had 36 inches.

Honey, I believe you're carrying that diet of yours too far. Heavens, 4 lbs. in a week are way too much. You're absolutely going to extremes.

What in the world has happened to the Chevy? You say the generator went bad. Gosh, I don't believe anything like that has ever happened before. Have you gotten it fixed yet? Don't forget Honey, those 12 gallons of A13 stamps must in some way be made use of by the 22nd of December.

P.S. Honey, I believe Mary (your cousin) wrote my address on that box of pretzels from Pomeroy's. If that was Mary you thank her very much for the Christmas gift. Enclosed I will send you the letter that was in the box.

[note enclosed]

At Holiday time our thoughts go out to our Fighting Forces wherever they might be with prayers for their safety and wellbeing, and most of all, our hopes for Victory and your safe, speedy return.

L.S. Hubbard-Managing Director

[Friday] December 15th

This morning I had to go to the Dental Clinic; I had another cavity which he filled. It was a real deep one but I think the Dentist did a good job. When I got back, I had to go get another injection for typhus fever.

This afternoon we had a two-hour lecture on how to unload weapons that our Infantry Unit uses. There are four in all so that if we find a wounded man on the field with his rifle, we must unload it.

Honey Bunch, I'm sending some things home; all my letters and some clothing which I have in excess. Please don't send any more Christmas gifts.

Dearest, Colorado is farther west than Texas but directly west of Pennsylvania. Gosh, I can't in the world understand why you don't get your mail more regularly. I send a letter away every day and yet you receive them at such irregular times.

So, the Transit Company workers of Reading went on strike. If you remember they had some difficulties already in the spring of this year but they averted a strike.

[Saturday] December 16th

What a day this has been. They are getting us ready to ship out and it looks as though we'll go for a long trip. This morning we were issued our mountain jackets and believe me those things really keep you warm. They have a hood attached to them you know which you put over your head. I also signed the payroll for December. At 10:00 AM we had a "Show Down" inspection. The officers came around and checked every piece of clothing and equipment we had. It all had to be placed on the bed in a certain manner too.

This afternoon was another headache. The whole barracks had to be scrubbed and washed. We had to move all the beds and equipment to ensure a good job. Then another order came through that we had to have our hair cut by 6:00 Monday morning. It had to be no more than 1 inch in length. I immediately went down to the barbershop and got them cut. By gosh, that barber cut them about 1/4 of an inch. Gee but I look funny. Ha! Ha! I look like a "cue ball" now. Maybe cutting them that short will help them grow. Ha! Ha!

Do you mean to tell me Honey that you don't have any money to do Christmas shopping?? Gosh, that's what I was afraid of, you run short and then can't buy the things you'd like to. Gee, you mustn't do that. Get money from the bank if that happens again.

Honey Darling, I'm not sending any cards (Christmas) to anybody except maybe in our family so you send them to my friends too. Of course, we sign both our names. Find out from Mother who I usually sent to. Honey, did you receive the box I sent you?? Now please don't open it before Christmas Day. Be a good girl.

Honey, how in the world did you get another cold? My, oh my, that worries me. Honestly, you must take better care of yourself. Now please don't lose so much weight and lower your resistance to the point where you can't fight off these cold germs.

[Sunday] December 17th

Today is Sunday and is just about the best day the Army has to offer. In fact, it's the best day in or out of the Army. I received a big box from Leesport. Gee whiz, they are all Christmas presents from Mother, Daddy, Grandma, and Sister. They were all wrapped in nice Christmas paper. Knowing that I won't be here for more than a few more days, I was forced to open them. There were socks, shirts, even a pencil and fountain pen[41], which I'm using. Yes, and the paper I'm writing on, they also sent me. I'm sending some of the things back home. I'm also sending my shoes (civilian) home. No person can realize how wonderful his folks are

---

[41] Fountain pens were being manufactured but still had to be filled with an ink bottle.

until we're not able to be together. It's just too bad I had to open all my presents before Christmas.

Dearest, you wanted to know about going to that Christmas dinner and party that the girls of your shop are having. Honey, I insist that you go. You don't get out enough. Please don't think for one moment that I object. I know my Dear will behave and act like a good wife, no matter who she's with.

Honey Bunch, I'm afraid you won't like very much what I have to say but I feel I should write it. Facts point toward us going to a POE Camp[42] from here. Yesterday we were told that starting Wednesday morning at 6:00 we'll be restricted to our area, we may not get in touch with anyone, etc. Our mail will be censured then etc. Things seem to be leading up to that. We were told that we may not have any visitors while at POE. I certainly hate to have to tell you this but you'll find it out soon anyway. Please don't let this worry you. Honestly, Darling, my biggest fear is not going overseas and the like but fearing that you people will worry and not enjoy your Christmas. Please, please don't worry. I'm very, very well and I'll take excellent care of myself.

Darling, don't tell anyone except our own family what I have to say. Under all probability, we're going to Virginia and then to Italy. This came from my 1st Sgt. He told me confidently. Even he might be wrong. Listen carefully, I won't be able to tell you where I'm in Virginia. Wait, I have a better idea, if I'm in the State of Virginia I'll put in my letter "Feed Judy well". If I'm in Maryland I'll write "Feed Nicky well". If I'm in New Jersey I'll write "Feed the general well". Do you understand that now?? Somewhere in my letter, I'll have those words. Indications point to us leaving Camp Swift

---

[42] Point of Embarkation Camps were staging areas to house and prepare troops for transport overseas.

sometime on Thursday. How long we'll be in POE I don't know but I think at least until January 1st. Dear, I've been as honest with you as I possibly can and now, I want a favor from you. I won't want this letter to sadden your Christmas. I'll be much closer to you by next Monday and we'll have a very good time dear because I'll follow your whole day of Christmas in my mind and that will make me very happy. You and Sister must brighten the day for both our parents. I wish both homes would have nice Christmas trees and enjoy the Christmas spirit. On Tuesday night, I believe we Protestants will have a Christmas Communion service before we leave Camp Swift. You see our chaplain will go overseas with us. That Testament that was among my gifts is certainly a nice present. That will come in handy. I have one now that was autographed by President Roosevelt. He tells you to read it faithfully.

[Christians received a pocket-sized volume of the New Testament and the Book of Psalms. A personal letter was written:

To the Members of the Army:

As Commander-in-Chief I take pleasure in commending the reading of the Bible to all who serve in the Armed Forces of the United States. Throughout the centuries, men of many faiths and diverse origins have found in the Sacred Book words of wisdom, counsel, and inspiration. It is a foundation of strength and now, as always, an aid in attaining the highest aspirations of the human soul.

Very sincerely yours,
Franklin D. Roosevelt

[Monday] December 18th

How is my wife? I hope she is fine. She seems to be somewhat depressed about the letter that I wrote home last

Wednesday. I have a confession to make, my Dear. Today I got a letter back that I had written you and low and behold it was last Friday's letter which you write you never received. I forgot to put on R.F.D. #2 and they directed it all over the city and then decided to return it to me. I'm sorry honey that I made that error.

Today I received three letters and eight Christmas cards. My Dear, I received 2 beautiful cards from my Wife. You sent me two Christmas cards Honey-two and they were so very nice. I'm not sure whether I want to send them home or not. I'd like so much to carry them with me. If they will let me keep them I will. However, I'd hate to lose them.

This afternoon we were talked to by our Regimental Commander Colonel Barlow. We're going to be in a parade tomorrow or Wednesday, the whole division, and pass in a review of the General.

Did you receive the Christmas present I sent you? Heavens you should be having it by now. It was mailed on Sunday.

Honey Darling, now please don't worry about where I'm going. It's not as bad as you might think. After all, there are millions of other American boys "over there" and I'm not any better than the next "GI Joe". As I said before, the chances seem to point to us going to Italy but really there is nothing certain.

Yes, Honey, I guess I'm as happy as a fellow can be without his loved ones. As I said before, I have no fear of going overseas or even of getting into combat.

[Tuesday] December 19th

Gosh, am I glad that today is over! It was the most hectic day I ever spent in the Army. About 8:15 I was awarded for my troubles, however. Well, let me attack the day from the time I got up.

I got up at the usual time, 5:45 AM. While I was brushing my teeth the 1st Sgt. came up to me and asked me if I was K.P. yet since I've been at Camp Swift. Well, I said I wasn't so I got the job. Ordinarily, I don't mind K.P. too much but today I did not want it. Today was the last day we had to mail our packages home and here I was on K.P. Well, I arranged to get off at 3 PM to go to the post office to mail it. Then to top it all off they told me at noon that I had 2 insured parcels to be picked up. Gosh alive, did that have me worried. Well, at 3 PM I went to get my packages, and here they were from my Darling. Gosh, I was at a loss to know what to do. Well, the one was pretty heavy and pretty securely wrapped so I decided to send it right back. The other was partially open so I decided on keeping it and hoping and praying I can keep everything that was in it. I don't know what was in the box I sent home but please my Dear, try to understand that it was the only thing I could do. Please, Darling, keep it for me until I get home. I was at the mess hall until 8 PM. That particular mess hall is closing up tonight and we had to clean up everything. Gosh, I never worked so hard in one day as I did today.

Well, Dear, when I got back to the barracks, I opened up your other package and Dear, I'm so glad I kept that one because I'm sure I'll be able to take everything with me. That bracelet you sent me is simply wonderful. My heart is filled with joy and appreciation. That "tree" is so cute also. That sweater Dear is just wonderful. I found out tonight that I can take it with me. It'll come in mighty handy in the Mountains. Words can't express how wonderful I feel since I opened up that box.

Honey Darling, I'll be traveling on the 18th train out of here for our next camp. Yes, some 20 full trains are leaving Camp Swift in the next three days with about 15-20 coaches on one train.

[Wednesday] December 20th

My Dear this will probably be a very short letter. By 4 PM all mail must be handed in. No more mail will be mailed until we get off the train at our next camp. We'll undoubtedly leave tomorrow sometime so don't expect any mail for a few days.

Today I got three packages, believe it or not. Fortunately, they are all food packages and the other fellows are helping me out in eating it. I'm saving some candy and cookies for our train ride. We're allowed to take such things with us on the train.

[Christmas card sent -To My Dear Wife at Christmas]
Do I wish you Merry Christmas?
Bless your heart, you know I do!
Everything that speaks of Christmas
Brings a loving thought of you,
For you are my "Christmas Spirit",
With your loving, thoughtful ways,
And I wish you all the blessings
You have brought to all my days. Luke

[Sunday] December 24th

How's everything in Berks? It's hard for me to write at all since our mail will be censored and I can't write all the things that are happening but you'll understand, I'm sure.

"It's the day before Christmas when all through the house, not a creature was stirring, not even a mouse." Do you remember that Christmas verse? Were you in Sunday School?? I hope so. I presume you and your Father will be going tonight and everybody will attend the dawn service tomorrow morning. I guess I won't be able to attend myself but I'm sure there'll be plenty in the future that we'll attend together. How about it??

How are all the animals coming along at home?? Is "Nicky's" leg any better?? Let's hope she stays off the street in the future. You must "feed Judy well" if you expect her to keep that girlish figure of hers!! Ha! Ha!

Dearest, I'm so hoping that you and all our families will have a very Merry, Merry Christmas.

[Monday] December 25th

A very Merry, Merry Christmas to all. How's the weather at home? Do you have a "White Christmas"?

I'm not sure I can tell you this but I hope they'll allow me to. We're along the Eastern Seaboard as you probably know. How long I'll be here I don't know. This morning another fellow and I went to church service at 10 AM. It did a fellow good to see all the soldiers that were at the service. They jammed the balcony and the choir pews. They even had chairs in the aisle. Then the chaplain announced at 11 AM there would be another service to take care of those that wouldn't get in the chapel. They even had a Public Address system connected for men on the outside. We sang lots of Christmas songs and hymns and had a fine Christmas Service.

I hope we'll have turkey for dinner. I understand we'll eat at 12:30. The mess halls are huge buildings and they really can feed lots of men in one sitting. The camp is quite a bit different than the one we just left. There are lots of trees and quite a lot of sand.

I've certainly been thinking about home today. I only hope and pray that all of you are having a Happy Time. Did you go back to your house after the dawn service? I take it that you'll eat your first dinner at your Grandparent's place and then go up home for another dinner at about 4 PM. Is that right? Now don't eat too much turkey but don't think of that shape of yours either. Christmas is one day we eat all we can. Ha! Ha!

You will be going to the Sunday School program then tonight also. Those small children always are so cute, aren't they??? Did your Sunday School class trim and decorate the church yesterday? Did you have a nice time on Wednesday night at this Christmas party you girls at the shop had? What present did you receive? I certainly hope you had a nice time. You must have more entertainment, my Dear.

I just got back from our Christmas dinner and believe me it was very good. We had turkey, bread filling, sweet potatoes, peas, cranberry sauce, apples, fruit salad, mince pie, and ice cream, and candy and nuts, and Hot Buns and butter.

How did you like that Christmas present I got you? Let's hope you like it?? Did all you people get your Christmas cards??

[Tuesday] December 26th

I must try and write smaller since I'll write on one side in case the censor does not like some of the things I'm writing. Gosh, Honey, I sure was glad to be able to talk to you yesterday. That really made our Christmas much happier. I just thought about calling around noon yesterday and I was determined to make the call no matter how long it would take.

Last evening after diner, I and a soldier from Philadelphia-a nice young chap- went to church service following which Holy Communion was held. The church was full again as it was in the morning. Yes, Ed is here too but he

105

isn't in the same barracks. He's two barracks down from where I'm residing.

[Wednesday]December 27th

They tell me that "Red" Skelton[43] is in camp for the last few days. He's appearing at some USO club. Tonight, I'm going to try and call home. Gosh, I wonder how long you're going to stay up at Leesport tonight?? Last night I put in a call at 8:10 PM and at 10 PM they told me it was a good 1 1/2 hour wait so I canceled it. I knew you'd be in bed by that time.

Honey Darling, the mail that you write me I understand will not be censored. They may "spot" censor it however, that is pick out a letter now and then from all incoming mail and look it over.

I told Ed about you wanting his girlfriend's address and he'll gladly give it to me. He thinks that would be a very good idea. Honey Bun, the bracelet fits beautifully. You absolutely couldn't have gotten me anything that I'd enjoy better. I can see it all the time and remember who gave it to me.

[Thursday] December 28th

I still didn't get any letter from you today. I believe the biggest mail call here is in the evening rather than at noon. So, I have high hopes of receiving 2 letters tonight. [Then there is a two-line cut out in the letter] Last night I received a letter from E.J. Poole, Vice President of Carpenter Steel Co. It was a nice letter wishing me a Merry Christmas and the like.

---

[43] A childhood actor who began in vaudeville during the 1930's and 40's who went on to radio, Broadway, movies and his own television show in 1951 called "The Red Skelton Show".

Boy, I was glad that I was able to get a call through last night and also very happy that I caught you there. Was it snowing very hard when your Father fetched you? Haven't you driven in the snow yet?? You must try it. It really is thrilling. Ha! Ha!

My Dear, you needn't worry about my birthday greeting or gift. You mustn't go to any excess trouble. I know you are wishing me a happy birthday.

My Darling, if you could only see me with this haircut of mine you would feel perfectly safe that no other woman would molest me. It's starting to grow a bit now but I still do not comb it so you can imagine how short it is.

Now listen Dear, in case you want to contact me in an extreme hurry as would be the case in an emergency we were told to tell you to notify your local chapter of the Red Cross. They can get in touch with me more quickly.

[Friday] December 29th

It started to snow now. Gosh, but it looks nice. I presume you think I'm still a child since I enjoy snow so much but I guess I'll never outgrow that. Ha! Ha!

We were given some instructions today as to the mailing of packages by people back home. I guess you know all the regulations by now. Any person can send one package a week to any particular soldier not to exceed five lbs. in weight or 15 inches in length.

You're getting my mail regularly, aren't you? We were told that it would not be delayed at all especially if we had nothing in it that had to be censored.

Dearest, I'm so very glad that you like your Christmas gift. Are you sure you like it as much as you say?? I was afraid you might not like the design. I'm also glad to hear you didn't open it until Christmas morning.

[Saturday] December 30th

Dearest, you sounded so very sleepy last night. I presume you weren't entirely awake, were you? I tried early enough in the evening to get you but the delay was about four hours. I was afraid you'd be in bed by that time. But it was so good to hear your voice again. I got them up home within a few minutes after I hung up our connection. Daddy was in bed but I was able to talk to everybody else.

Dear, I'm so glad that Mother is taking things so very well. With everything she has on her mind, she is a courageous woman. I only hope she continues to stay that way.

Gosh, I'm sorry that I didn't keep that other box of yours. Those cookies and cashew nuts hit the spot with me. Well, I'll have to ask you to send some of them sometime in the future if you don't mind.

[Sunday] December 31st

My gosh, I can hardly believe that this year is just about at the end. We usually went to see a movie on New Year's Eve, didn't we? Well, this year will be a little different but don't worry those happy days will be forthcoming I'm sure.

As you probably have guessed, I'm writing this letter at the telephone "center". I've been here since 1:25 PM. I got my calls placed at 2 PM. When they will start coming through is a problem. The place is jammed with soldiers.

Yes, My Dear, there are WACS stationed here-quite a few it seems but you don't have to worry in the least about me. I'm a very bashful boy and then too, I'm strictly a one-woman man. Ha! Ha! From what little I've seen of the WACS they are a homely bunch of old maids. Of course, maybe my eyes don't notice their beauty. Well, no one can come up to my Dear Wife.

Ruth, you must do something about your eye. Now you promised me for a long time you'd go to a doctor about it and you seem not to go. My heaven, you've left that thing drag long enough.

This morning at 10 AM I went to Church Service. I've never seen so many soldiers attend services as I do here. It might be the thought of what might be ahead for them- what the future has in store.

Honey, you said in a letter that I'd have a large bank account when I get back. Dear, that money is yours as much as it is mine and don't forget to use it if ever the occasion arises. I'll be getting a $25 bond a month now but maybe we should buy some whenever we get some extra money saved. They are good investments. Use your judgment.

[Monday] January 1st, 1945

Ruth Dear, I was hoping and praying I'd never have to hear the news you wrote. It just doesn't seem possible that such a thing can be possible. Honey, I can perfectly understand why you didn't want to tell me the news over the telephone. I also can now see why you seemed a bit different on Friday and Sunday when I called, and yet, Honey, you tried so hard to make things seem right. Howard was my brother-in-law. I certainly didn't know him as his sister and parents did yet I knew him well enough to respect him very highly. He was just the finest young man one could know. His habits were the best, and he was indeed representative of the finest type of American manhood. It was a privilege to know him. I can imagine how difficult it must be for you and your parents. I only wish there was something I could do to help. If there is anything I can do, please tell me. As the New Year dawns, we can only pray that this terrible conflict will soon come to an end. When I think of Howard, of how he lived and died, I am reminded of the great biblical quotation "Greater Love Hath No Man Than This, That He Lay Down His Life For His Friend". Well, Dear, as your Grandfather said, "he's better off than we are". We know where he is now so we must rest our minds and hearts and face the world anew.[44]

Gosh, My Darling, no matter how long it takes to get you on the phone, it indeed is worth it. I feel as though I can not only hear you but also see you. I'm glad I was able to talk to your parents. My heart bleeds for both of them as well as for my Dear Wife. I only wish there was something I could do to help them.

Yes, Dearest, I'm so glad that you and Sister went to a movie last Thursday. You must go more often. You always enjoyed movies so very much, Honey, so I want you to go.

Dearest, that Birthday card you sent me was so very beautiful. Your parents, too, sent me such a nice Birthday greeting. They are so very kind to me. We're so lucky to have such great parents, aren't we Ruth??

[Tuesday] January 2nd

It was an extremely lovely day. The weather was cold but it was nice and clear. I still can't enjoy any snow yet. Let's hope that I'll see some before the winter is over. Are you still having snow up home?

My Dear, you and Sister seem as though you two just can't lose at the game of Rook. You must give Grandma and Mother an advantage. Give them about 100 or 150 to start with. Then they might be able to win. How about it? Ha! Ha! Ha!

---

[44] Howard Kunkleman was updated from missing to "killed in action" and is buried in the National Cemetery in Gettysburg, Pa.

Dearest, you got very nice gifts for Christmas. All that Fostoria[45] ware you received is very useful. That was mighty nice of your Grandfather to give you all that money. Now please use it for anything you wish. So, you have our picture in your locket. Gosh, that's all right. I knew it opened but I didn't know you wanted to put anything in it.

What does your cousin Donald do in the Merchant Marine?[46] Is he a cook or does he do something else?

Yes, my Dearest, I know you'll be the same good woman when I get back that you are now but you must go to the movies or go with your friends sometimes. You don't get enough entertainment, my Dear.

Yes, I wish I could be with you people when you eat all that meat that you got from the "pig". That is a very economic idea to buy meat that way. There are so many kinds of meat cuts that a person can get.

I can hardly believe that a husband can be as mean to his wife as Mr. "M" is. Do you mean to tell me that he asked her to leave?? Gosh, I can hardly believe that such things can exist. To think that he doesn't give her enough money for food is unbelievable. What they should do with a fellow like that is put him on the front lines. Anybody that makes people that miserable should get what he deserves.

---

[45] The Fostoria Glass Co. located in Fostoria, Ohio began manufacturing in 1887 and lasted about 100 years. They made stemware, container glass and dinner ware in many different colors.

[46] The Merchant Marine was made up of civilian and federally owned merchant ships that transported soldiers and war equipment to aid the war effort.

Deployed to Northern Italy

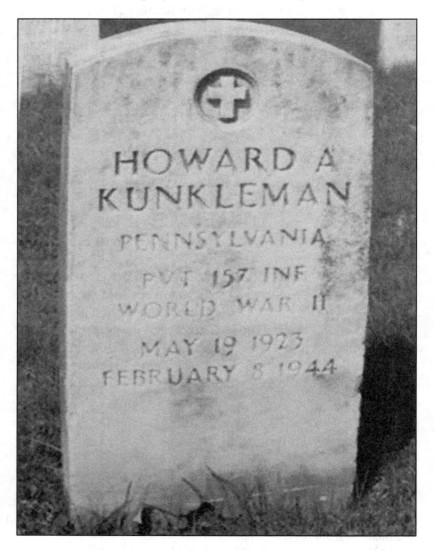

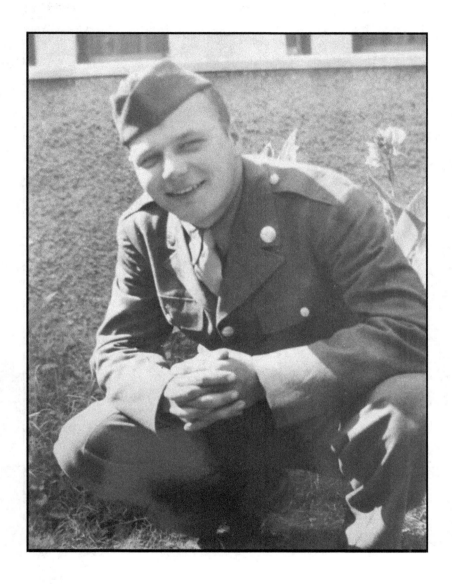

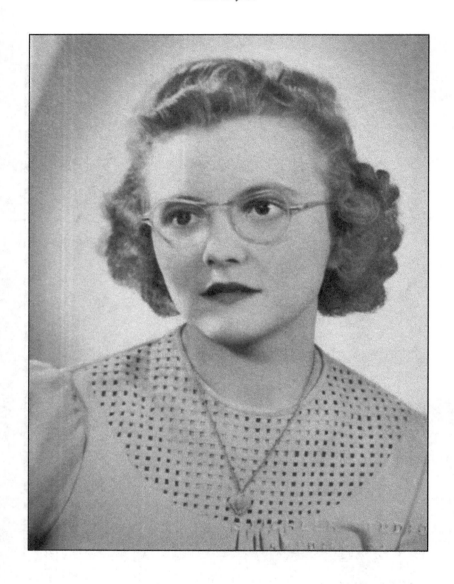

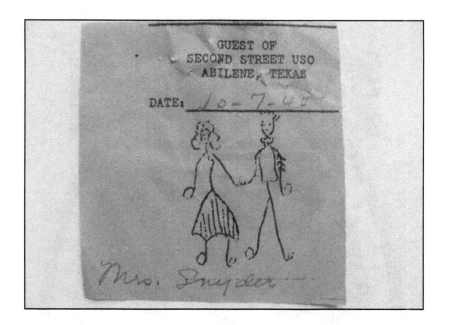

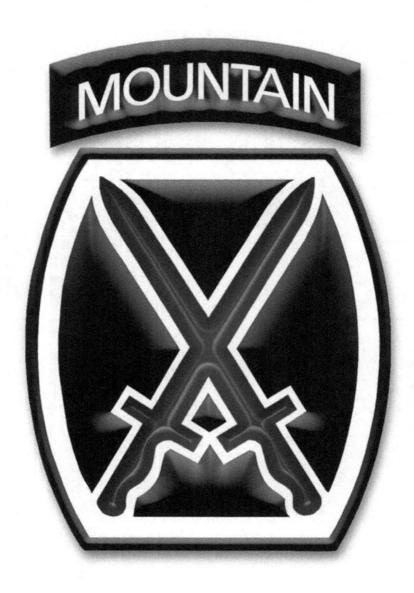

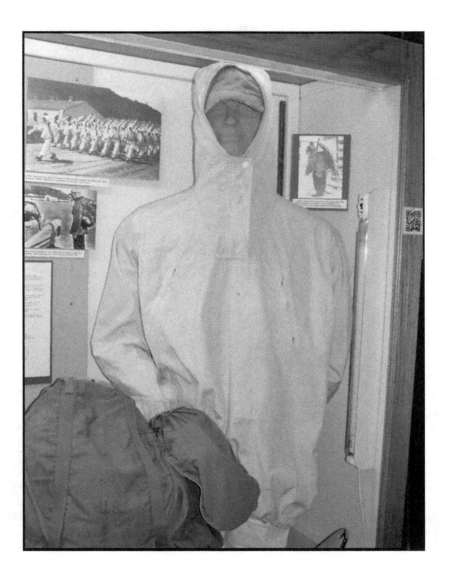

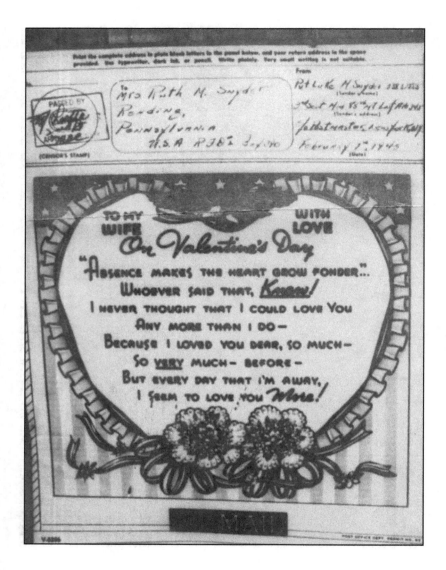

Leesport Medic Cited for Heroism On Italian Front

Pfc. Luke M. Snyder, first eschlon medical corpsman attached to the Tenth Mountain Division, has been awarded the Bronze Star Medal for "heroic achievement" in action on April 15, near Castle d'Aiano, Italy. The action for which the citation is given occurred in the strongly-defended mountainous area south of Bologna on the second day of the drive which pushed the Germans out of Italy.

During two days of strenuous fighting, the strength of Company I was reduced from 199 men to 46, 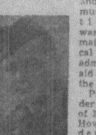 and during much of this time Snyder was the only remaining medical personnel to administer first aid and bring in the wounded.

Private Snyder is the son of Mr. and Mrs. Howard C. Snyder, Leesport, and is the husband of the former Ruth Kunkelman, Reading R. D. 2. He

Luke Snyder

is a graduate of Ursinus College and prior to entering the service was employed by the Carpenter Steel Company.

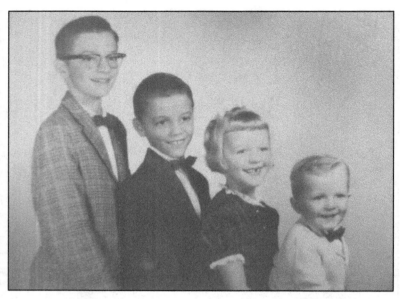

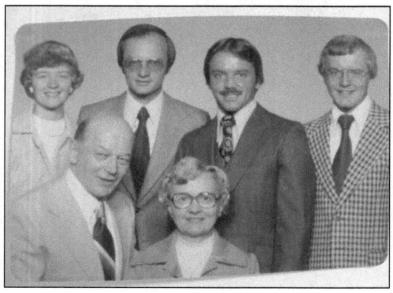

[Monday] January 8th

I had plans of writing a little note every day but this doggone ocean had something to say about the whole matter. Ha! Ha! After one day out, I felt like I do when I used to go on a "Merry-Go-Round". The only place that I feel half decent is in my bunk but I've decided that I must try and write a few lines.

When we left Camp the Camp Band was there to see us off. You know it was one of those old-fashioned "going away" concerts with all the marches that I always enjoyed. Of course, under the circumstances, they didn't quite sound like they did when I used to play them in the Centerport Band. Ha! Ha!

The last letter I received from my Dear was the one she wrote on Friday the 29th. I also received four birthday cards from the folks up home, they were all very pretty. One of them contained a $5.00 bill.

The ship we're on is quite a large one. More than that I cannot tell you. When we pulled out of the harbor, the bands were again playing. It gives a fellow a funny feeling when he pulls away from this good old U.S.A. not knowing exactly when he'll return.

[Tuesday] January 9th

Another day has dawned. I feel better than I did for the last few days so while I feel up to it, I'll have to pen a few lines. Since we've last seen land, I've moved my watch up two hours so now you people have but 10 AM instead of Noon. I'll probably have to move it up again a few more hours until we reach our destination.

We eat but twice a day on-board ship and I can easily see why. They'd be feeding us from 6 AM until midnight if we'd get three meals a day. The Deck, of which I am a part, eats about 8:30 and then again about 5 PM. That is, we get in line about those times. Till we finally get to the mess hall an extra hour lapses, so you can imagine how long it takes to feed everybody on board. I haven't been going to many of the meals lately because the doggone rocking makes me feel too light-headed. Ha! Ha! But don't you worry, Darling. I'm O.K.

I was on Deck this morning and it's a beautiful day. The sky is clear and the ocean blue. It's really a beautiful sight. If only my Darling was with me and we'd be crossing on a huge luxury liner. Wouldn't that be wonderful, Dear?

I'm glad, Honey, you went to work last Friday. I guess you didn't feel like it but it doesn't help sitting around and thinking about things. If only there was something I could do to help matters but I'm so helpless.

Gosh, but I wish I could see that picture you just put in your locket. I believe it's a beauty. Yes, it helped to get your Mother's mind off of unpleasant thoughts. Do you like the locket so much you're wearing it every day???

The Red Cross brought around a small "shaving" bag which contained a "Pocket Book", a deck of cards, a pencil, paper, and the like.

[Thursday] January 11th

We are now four hours up since we left the good old U.S.A. Today I feel better than I have as yet on the whole trip. I guess it's because the ocean is calmer today.

I didn't go to breakfast this morning but I went to supper. We had good stew, spaghetti, bread and jelly, cakes, and cocoa. Gosh, I was surprised we had cocoa instead of coffee. I had something to drink for a change. Yesterday I hadn't gone to any of the meals because I wasn't feeling up to it. It's amazing how little food a fellow can get along on.

Are your parents all right?? Are they taking things as well as can be expected?? It just seems as though such things can't happen.

Whatever I write on board ship will be mailed when we dock, so there'll be letters on the way as soon as possible.

[Friday] January 12th

I decided, Honey, to write a V-Mail[47] letter for a change. Once I get situated and can write regularly, I'll write and mail at the same time an Air Mail and V-Mail letter and we'll see which one you'll receive first.

This afternoon I was up on Deck and they had an orchestra playing for about an hour.

Gee Whiz but I love my Darling. Are you behaving yourself? Ha! Ha! Just kidding, you know.

[Saturday] January 13th

This morning for breakfast we had a couple of hard-boiled eggs, some cream of wheat, two apples, potatoes, bread and butter, and some cake. It was a real good breakfast.

I didn't do much the whole day. This morning it was beautiful on Deck! The sky was cloudless. Then at noon, it started getting cloudy and by 2 PM it was pouring down raining. For a few minutes, it was hailing.

My Darling, do you know what, we won't get to see any hockey games this season or for that matter any basketball games at Northwest either. How is Hershey doing by this time? You must write and tell me how the Bears are making

---

[47] Soldiers wrote letters on special limited space sheets which were a combined letter and envelope. These were reduced to thumbnail size on microfilm rolls and sent to designated areas in the U.S. where they were censored and reproduced to a 4x5 inch letter that was sent to the recipient. This saved space and weight for overseas shipping.

out. They were in second place the last I saw with Buffalo in First. How is Albright doing? They won their first three games, I know, but I haven't seen any late results.

My Dear, I was quite right when I gave you a hint as to where I was going. Do you know now where I am? It seems as though I'm following Howard around although I've come here directly.

Whatever you are wishing for
That's what I'm wishing too!
To give you happiness is part
Of all, I plan to do.
And not just on this day, my Dear,
 But always my life be
Filled with all the happiness
That you have brought to me.

Yes, My Darling, that was the beautiful reading from the birthday greeting you sent to me and that's just what I'm wishing you too.

[Wednesday] January 17th (Somewhere in Italy)

Please, My Dear, don't be angry with me since I didn't write for a few days. I just didn't have the opportunity. Just kidding. Ha! Ha! It's amazing how little time a fellow receives to write letters. The time just doesn't arrive. Well, as you can see by my heading I'm somewhere in Italy, where I cannot tell you. On the trip over we passed the Rock of Gibraltar[48] which was an interesting sight to see. We've read and studied so much about it and now I've actually seen it. Only one night was the ocean quite wild and I was told that even that wasn't very bad but being a newcomer on the ocean

---

[48] A large limestone rock that juts out into the Straits of Gibraltar from the southern coast of Spain.

it seemed rough to me. The liner we came over on was a beauty. We made the trip in a comparatively short time.

Well, I've now felt my foot on foreign soil. Ha! Ha! This is Italy where I was told olive trees would grow and the whole country was as it was termed "Sunny Italy". Well, hereafter don't believe anything like that until you can see for yourself for the weather is rather chilly. This morning we had a real thick frost but now the sun has come out and it is warming up. For the time at least we're pitching our pup tents and I'm very fortunate in having a fire right in front of our tent. Of course, it usually means that you'll have to get the wood to keep it going but that's O.K. by me.

A very unfortunate condition exists here in Italy. People come up along the road and stand around, hoping you'll give them some food or old clothing. They'll do anything for some cans of "C" or "K" rations[49] and we soldiers complain when we have to eat them. Yes, they're luxuries to the Italians. Do you remember all those newsreels we saw in the movies of how the places were bombed? Well, I've seen enough to collaborate with all those pictures. The country has really taken a beating! What irks me about the way they do things in the U.S.A. when I see all the trees that line the highways here in Italy. I have not seen too much yet but large trees (spruce I believe) line both sides of the street and form sort of an archway across the road. Gosh, I believe in the spring of the year it would be beautiful. Over in the States, they cut all the trees down whether they have to or not.

---

[49] These were canned food they carried that could be eaten hot or cold when troops were cut off from base camp. The main meal was basically meat with either beans, spaghetti or vegetables. The labels were known to come off so it became a mystery meal. Bread and desserts were also canned. They were provided with coffee, sugar, salt. powdered lemon or lime juice, cocoa powder and hard candy.

I still didn't receive any mail from the states. I guess it'll still be quite a few days until any begins arriving. Boy, I'll be in my glory when all those letters start coming. I just heard a rumor that some of the mail is in the vicinity. Let's hope that's true. Gosh, my pocketbook is certainly being used a lot just taking your picture out and gazing at it.

[Thursday] January 18th [Italian money enclosed]

I'm having the opportunity the last two mornings to write early so I'm doing it. At night I would be forced to write by candle and that isn't nearly as proficient as by sunlight. We had another heavy frost this morning. I had forgotten to tell you on our trip over we passed the Isles of Capri.[50] That's quite a famous island. I also saw Mt. Vesuvius, that renowned volcano. She seems rather quiet now, however. My Darling, if I'd like wine, I certainly could get plenty of it here. The Italians seem to have plenty of that and exchange it willingly for food or tobacco of some sort.

[Friday] January 19th

You are sleeping soundly right now Honey. How about it? This is the first undesirable day we've had since we're in Italy. At about 5 AM I woke up and the rain was really coming down. I fetched in all my belongings, put them in the tent, and went back to sleep. The wind is pretty strong. Let's hope our pup tent stands the test.

My Darling, some of my interests have already. been aroused. You know how interested I am in various types of money, how I watch every piece of money that passes through my fingers. Well, our money has been exchanged for

---

[50] Located on the south side of the Gulf of Naples, it's noted for its beautiful blue water, steep rocky hills that project above the sea with houses of different colors on the hillside.

what is known as "Allied Military Currency". This money we cannot take out of the country but the money that was formerly used by the Italians, of course, is no longer of any value. Yesterday I exchanged a pack of cigarettes to an Italian for four pieces of their former paper money. These are "Lire" notes and right now 1 Lire corresponds to 1 penny in American money. I have one 10 Lire, 1 Five Lire, one 2 Lire, and one 1 Lire. I think I'll enclose two of these notes in this letter and the other two in a future letter so that in case one of the letters fail to reach you, you'll at least have seen some of their money.

I still haven't any mail from Berks County. Be sure, my Dear, you let me know immediately if you receive any further news regarding Howard's status. I'm so anxious to know if anything different has taken place.

I heard this morning that the war news is rather favorable for our side. Let's hope it continues as such and that victory is not too far distant. It really is a fact that back home in the states one knew more about how things were going than one does here.

[Sunday] January 21st

How are you this beautiful Sunday morning? I guess you're still sleeping soundly while we are having noon hour already. I still haven't gotten any mail from home since we left the states but I have high hopes of getting some soon. Yesterday I wasn't able to write. Please forgive me I just didn't get a single minute in which to pen a few lines. You must not worry if you fail to hear from me for some days.

Well, My Dear, they've had some changes made and I've finally encountered my wish. Ha! Ha! Yes, we're having quite a bit of snow. Where I am last night, we had a real blizzard.

Temperatures hit sub-zero every night. We're in buildings now, no more tents.

[Monday] January 22nd [stamped "Reading Feb 20, 1945"- Pa. plus "Passed by Army Examiner" stamp]

We still haven't received any mail from home but I understand that within a day or two we might have some coming our way. There'll be a happy time among us when that time comes. I guess you're wondering why I haven't requested anything yet? Gosh, but it slips my mind every time I write. You can send me some cookies, candy, and gum, pretzels and potato chips. Last night for chow we had what they called "Vienna Sausages", salmon, cookies, and chocolate pudding. It was all very good.

How are your parents, my Dear? Whenever I write to you, I also am writing to them. You understand, don't you? Is Daddy holding up O.K.?? Gosh, I'm so afraid he'll just sit and worry, worry, worry. Every time you see him impress upon his mind that I'm O.K.

When I think of you and how much we mean to each other it makes all these days pass more quickly and the time when we'll be together again closer.

[Tuesday] January 23rd

Yesterday after finishing your letter and while writing home to Leesport we had our first mail call since "way back when" and I was very lucky for I received a letter from My Dear Wife. It was the one you wrote on Jan. 2nd. Gee, but I can't tell you often enough how much I appreciated that letter.

My Darling, we're living in a small Italian Mountain Village and we're living in abandoned Italian homes. I'm writing this by the light of a candle so if you can't understand my writing you'll understand.

[Wednesday] January 24th

This morning when I got up the fellows that sleep in the same room as I do, said there was mail call last night at about 10:30 and there was lots of mail for me. I had gone to bed before that time and they didn't want to wake me. Gee, I wish they would have but as it was, I received seven letters this morning. I've read the letters twice by this time.

Gosh, but I was hungry this noon. I could have eaten a "dozen" meals, I believe. We had beef hash, spaghetti and sauce, sauerkraut, and cooked apples. It was a real good meal.

My Dear, I understand perfectly why you never mentioned anything about Howard over the phone. That was perfectly all right. I guess I can understand too why you didn't go to Sunday School on the 31st but if I were you, I would go hereafter. I feel that a person finds comfort in going to church and Sunday School at moments when our heart is heavy. I know people ask a lot of questions but they mean it well.

Yes, Virginia's husband was very fortunate to get home from his P.O.E. but it just doesn't happen that way for everybody. Don't worry, My Dear, our day will come and we'll just celebrate that much more. How about it???

Honey, you must wear that black velvet dress when it's finished, have someone take a picture of you and send it to me. All kidding aside, if you can get films have some pictures taken and send them. This is no order, just a suggestion. Ha! Ha! Ha!

Gosh, I must laugh when I think of you buying an Ouija Board.[51] Yes, I've heard about them before but I never had

---

[51] This was a flat board with letters, numbers and the words "yes", "no" and "Goodbye" printed on it. Game players would place their fingers on the heart shaped piece of plastic or wood and when a question was asked the piece was said to be possessed by the spirit of a person and would

too much faith in them. I personally think they're a lot of "hooey" but lots of people have quite a bit of faith in them. It's interesting though to see what they have to say.

[Thursday] January 25th

During the night we had more snow and it really looks pretty. It was wet snow and it clung to all the trees.

I believe I forgot to tell you a couple of days ago I bandaged a fellow soldier's leg and we got talking and lo and behold he was from Reading. He went to Southwest Junior High where Father was principal and to Rose and Washington Grade School where I had gone for six weeks when I was in the sixth grade. He remembered me very well. I can't say that I knew him. Wasn't that a coincidence though???

I'm so glad that your Mother enjoys making "jigsaws". It'll help take her mind off unpleasant thoughts. The best thing one can do is keep yourself busy. When you have made those two that you have you can get plenty more up home.

Yes, Darling, don't you worry-speaking of V. Bowman and her baby, our time will come. We'll have everything and will be so very happy together.

[Friday] January 26th

Last night, Honey Bunch, a couple of fellows, and I walked through the village we're staying in and encountered a rather elderly Italian who invited us to his house. One of the soldiers among us could speak Italian so we decided to go with him. He had a wife and two children. Honey Dear, you should see how these Italians are living. They have a form of electricity that produces such a very dim light that it hardly has any value. The candles we use have more power than

---

move on its own to answer or spell out a response. This became popular in the 19th century and continued into the 1960's.

their electric light, so you can imagine how much light they throw. He was telling us about how the Germans had treated them. They had tied him to a post and whipped him. His wife was sick at the time. They took all the clothing they had, even made the children strip. For people like that, one must really feel sorry. You should have heard what the husband had to say about "our friend" Mussolini.[52] My, how he hates him. They would so much like to come to America after the war. Some of these Italians I certainly am in sympathy with but there are some that I wouldn't trust further than I could see them, especially the younger men.

I just happened to get a hold of a paper; "The Stars and Stripes"[53] which is published here in Italy for us soldiers. I see where Hershey is still in second place in the Eastern League with Buffalo in first, six points ahead. Are you still watching all the sports news? I also saw when Albright beat a Mexican team of a sort. How are they doing anyway?? My Darling, you must go to some basketball and hockey games. I'm sure you can find someone that would like to go.

Did your parents decide to write that address which they received to acquire some information about Howard? Gee, I think they absolutely should write. I'm sure that if they don't, they'll wish they had later.

My Darling, so far, I've been plenty warm. In case I ever need my scarf I'll send for it. Don't worry, Darling about me being cold.

---

[52] He was the prime Minister of Italy from 1922 until 1943 where at that time he'd become a dictator of Italy. He then became the leader of the Italian Social Republic which was attached to German control in Northern Italy. In April of 1945 he tried to escape, was captured and later executed.
[53] This newspaper began being printed during the Civil War in Bloomfield, Missouri. During World War II the newspaper gave real time information to the troops in several operating theaters and is still in current publication today.

[Sunday] January 28th

My Dear, I've moved to a new location. Temperatures remain about the same. The town we're in now is larger than the one we had been in the last few days. The people, as a rule, seem to be better off.

Say, Dear, did you get around to paying my church dues for the remainder of 1944?

This morning, Dear, I met another fellow from Reading. Isn't that a coincidence?? He lives on Mulberry Street. When I told him where I was from, he said I probably knew "Ray" who runs that hotel above Dauberville. I said I did. Do you know where I mean? I'm sure your Father knows him too. Well, this soldier is this Ray's brother-in-law. When I told him my name, he looked at me more closely and said "I've seen you before". Here I found he worked at the Standard Auto Body Works above Reading. We've often had our dents taken out of our cars there. It's the place your Father had his car fixed when Howard had the accident and we went down for it. Isn't that something? Ha! Ha! It seems that no matter where you go, even in Italy, you'll meet some people from home.

So, Sister's room is still very hot, even in the middle of the winter. And she always likes a lot of covers, too. Doesn't she?? Poor you! Ha! Ha! You must kid her about you attempting to "choke" her. That's a laugh. Now I know why I almost suffocated some nights. Ha! Ha! I guess you were trying to choke me. Aren't you ashamed?? Ha! Ha!

[Monday] January 29th

Gosh, no matter what a fellow does or how he feels when he writes to his Dear, Wife, he feels 100% better. My Darling you must remember the night of January 27th, 1945.[54] Don't

---

[54] On this date the Red Army liberated inmates of the Auschwitz-Birkenau concentration camp in Poland.

forget to remind me to tell you. What happened on that night it seems as one's whole life is filled with new experiences.

How's my Darling Wife behaving?? Just kidding. I'm sure she's a very, very good girl.

[Tuesday] January 30th

Well, our President is celebrating his birthday. How old is he anyway? He must be pretty high in the '60s, isn't he?? This is a great day for the Warm Springs Institution for Infantile Paralysis.[55] That is a dread disease when it attacks an individual.

Dearest, I've moved again. I'm in another small village. I've certainly moved many times since I've hit the shores of Italy. Holy Smokes, doesn't the time fly. I wish it would fly right on until it's time for us to head back to the U.S.A., how about it?? Of course, maybe my Dear doesn't want me back anymore. Ha! Ha! Just kidding!

Say, you mentioned being able to send me a box of Hershey chocolate bars.[56] Gosh, that will be just fine. I'm requesting that box right now if it's not too much trouble on your part. Send any kind you can get. My preference is the Almond Bar, but any will do.

Gosh, my Dear, I'm glad you started our Christmas funds again. Gee, that'll cost you $2.00 a week. That's quite a bit. Listen, Darling, you use that extra $25 that I gave you from

---

[55] Franklin Roosevelt visited Warm Springs, Georgia in 1924 in hopes of benefiting from the thermal springs. He purchased a rundown resort there in 1927 and made it into what today is a well-known rehabilitation center focusing on hydrotherapy treatments.

[56] This company located in Hershey. Pa was founded by Milton S. Hershey in 1894. It began mass producing its "Hershey Bar" in 1905. He introduced the "Hershey Kiss" in 1907. In 1942 this production was interrupted due to rationing aluminum foil. This part of the plant was converted to make chocolate paste for the soldiers.

my Christmas fund. You see I took $25 when I left home. I owe you $50 anyway. Remember you gave me that at Abilene. I still owe you $25. No, my Darling, our bank account isn't bad at all. I only hope you'll not economize too much. My Dear, if you get any money on hand, why you can buy a small bond. The government needs the money all right and it is a good investment. In your itemized expenditures of the 10th, you had a car bill of $360. Was that for the Chevy?? When you had Stoudt work on it?? Yes, your hubby isn't earning too much these days. He's very sorry but someday he'll do better. Is he forgiven?? Ha! Ha! Ha!

You people sure do put those jigsaw puzzles together in a hurry. Yes, I'm very glad that you like to make them. I could never stay at them for too long a time. Right now, I'm alternating between V-Mail and Air Mail. Which comes through the fastest? Numbering your letters is a very good idea. I usually get at least two or three letters at one time so that will be a great help.

[Wednesday] January 31st
When a fellow looks over the snowcapped mountains with the sun shining brightly it is a beautiful sight.

[Thursday] February 1st
Gee, we're living in style lately! This noon we had French fried potatoes. The kitchen we're connected with now is feeding only 18 men and they make good food. It seems we eat with a different group every few days.

I haven't seen "Ed" for about three weeks and I have no idea when I'll get to see him. I'm anxious to know how he's getting along.

Yes, my Dear, I feel exactly the way you do about Howard. It seems terrifically funny that all of a sudden, they say he was killed almost a year ago, and yet at that time they had no way of telling what had happened to him. Don't think that the telegram is absolutely right. It might be of course and it also might turn out entirely differently. We must hope and pray for the best. I'm sure things will work out all right.

Dearest, you get something real nice from that Christmas money you received, anything at all. If you need a raincoat be sure and get one. You have that red one right now, do you not? Honey, I still remember what you have even though I haven't seen it for a few months. Ha! Ha! You're also speaking of shoes. Why don't you buy shoes with that money?? Do you still need ration stamps for shoes??

Honey, you see I didn't receive the letters you wrote on the 6th and 7th of the month, so I hadn't known that you were ill until I received the letter of the 11th when you found out you must have had the "48-hour flu". Are you alright now? It seems my whole family has something the matter with them. How about it?

[Friday] February 2nd

So, you're looking for souvenirs from Italy?? Dearest, do you think I'm over here on my leisure time? Ha! Ha! So far, I haven't been able to come across anything but if I do, I'll send some home or tell the people to reserve them and you and I will come back after the war for them. How about that?? We're going to do some traveling, aren't we Honey Bunch?? Of course, I guess we better see more of the U.S.A. before we see foreign lands.

My Dearest, it's absolutely impossible for me to secure any Valentine's greetings this year but with this letter, I'm sending you all the love and good wishes that Valentine's Day brings.

[Saturday] February 3rd

My Dearest isn't up yet this Saturday morning and her husband put in 4 hours of hard work already. Gosh, I forgot to tell you two days ago we got paid. By gosh we even get paid out here in no-man's land. I hit the jackpot. I received $22.20. You see they only took out $7.50 for a bond whereas starting with February they'll take out $18.75. That's why I received so "much" money. I'm very sorry your husband doesn't have a better job but someday I'll be able to make a little more money. Ha! Ha!

Dearest, you mustn't get mad at your manager because of what she does in her private life. That's really her own business. Naturally what she does is not the right thing but just let her carry on. I guess she told you when she said "you're behind the times". I never knew that one was behind the times when one didn't run around with other men or women. That's a new one on me. How about it? Yes, my darling, I guess I can't be sure of you now not falling in love with another man. Ha! Ha!

Gee whiz, I believe when I get to a shower or bath, I'll stay in it for about six hours. I haven't had a decent wash since I left our ship.

Ruth, I'm so glad your parents are taking everything so well. It's not easy, believe me, there really is nothing one can do. So, you're still wearing your locket every day. My, but you must like it! I hope I didn't make too bad a selection. I didn't have too much time picking it so I wasn't sure it was what you'd like.

Yes, My Dear, the way it looks I failed to do my stuff. But I can't see why it's always my fault. Ha! Ha! They always say it takes two to pick a fight. Well, I presume that goes in this case too. Ha! Ha! Well, don't worry, when I get back things are going to "pop" and I mean pop. I'm really going to make "hay".

I see Albright lost to Muhlenberg the other night. Gosh, Muhlenberg must have another crack team this year. I consider them on par with the best in the country.

[Sunday] February 4th

Honey, Darling, tonight I'm extremely tired, I doubt that I was as tired as I am now, but I must write my daily letter to my dearest wife. Honey the last 24hours I've experienced something that I never thought I'd ever see or live through and tonight I'm a mighty thankful man that I'm able to write this letter. It's been some time since I last grabbed some sleep so I'll hit the hay as soon as I'm finished writing. Nobody ever has to tell me that I'm not well physically outside of being tired I'm very well and feeling fine

Dearest, you go right ahead and get your permanent wave, and Honey Bunch you wear your hair any way at all.

[Monday] February 5th

Gosh, but I enjoy reading your mail. It makes a fellow feel so very, very good. Honey, thanks too for sending the clipping from the Eagle. It's interesting to read about what's happening back home. Yes, I believe spring is coming to Italy a bit early this year. I feel quite good today after a good night's sleep. When I get home, I'm telling you a lot more about what happened and where I was. A man experiences quite a few things in war, I'm sure.

A few days ago, I met a fellow from Topton, Pa. I can't remember his name anymore but "boy" did he have a "Dutch" accent. Of course, it certainly did remind me of home.

Well, my dear, did you ask for a raise?? You were telling me about one of the girls getting more money if she'd stay? It seems that nobody is getting along with that manager you have.

How's your "green" Fascinator[57]coming along? Is your Mother making you one?? I think they are very nice "headgear" if I may call them as such. I never got those cards from Carpenter Steel yet. I presume that is when they do come it'll be a straight deck. I'll probably play solitaire with them.

Yes, Honey, I've got your picture right with me all the time. I have it in my pocket with my pay-book rather than in my wallet.

[Tuesday] February 6th

This morning I'm in another town again. The snow has melted quite a bit and it's muddy and slushy. I still am missing about six or seven letters from earlier in the month. Gosh, but I enjoy reading your letters. I was still reading last night after everyone else had gone to sleep.

[Wednesday] February 7th (a printed V-Mail in the shape of a heart)

To My Wife with Love, on Valentine's Day
"Absence makes the heart grow fonder"
Whoever said that, Knows!
I never thought that I could Love You
Any more than I do-
Because I love you, Dear, so much-

---

[57] This described a headpiece usually made of lightweight knitted fabric, sometimes tied under the chin. During the war hats were classified as a luxury and taxed at 33 % so many women took to making their own.

so very much- before
But every day that I'm away, I seem to love you MORE!

[Wednesday] February 7th

Gosh, my Dear is very thoughtful. Yesterday I received two very beautiful Valentine greetings from her. Yesterday I also received those cards from the Carpenter Steel Co. They are expensive cards. There are two decks put together as "partners" if you know what I mean. I must use them but I don't know what to play. Many would use them, however, if I'd want to give them up.

This morning we received some "PX" rations including six pieces of candy, some cookies, and some hard candy. Speaking of requests, it seems somewhat difficult to acquire soap and toothpaste. You can send me some of those if you think of it.

Another beautiful day. It's clear and the sun is nice and warm. By the way, I also received a copy of that newspaper "Reading Newsweek". Carpenter Steel sends it to all their men in the Armed Services. It was the issue of December 19th and on the front page, there was a huge picture of Penn Street taken during that four-day trolley and bus strike. There wasn't a single bus or trolley on the street except that "Trailways" bus parked in front of Witners, the one owned by the Allentown and Reading Transit Co. What a sight!!!

Honey, did you receive any further news from the War Dept. as to what they think happened to Howard? Gosh, please inform me the moment you hear anything in regards to the matter.

Yes, that's a mighty fine organization to belong to, My Dear-the Eastern Star. It's a woman's lodge much like the Masons is a man's lodge. You join it before I get back if you wish.

Has Rachael heard from Earl yet? Have the Rothenbergers heard more from Eugene?? When a man is missing at sea, I think there's more reason to be alarmed than he's missing on land.

Yes, my Dear, August 23rd, 1939 was absolutely the biggest day in my life. It's one I'll never, never forget. I believe the next biggest day of my life will be when I see my Honey again. Gosh, I think of that day so very much.

How's Ontelaunee making out in basketball? I presume they're losing again this year as usual.

[Thursday] February 8th

My Dear, the letter you wrote after you got back from the Doctor really worries me. How in the world could you ever have paralyzed a nerve in your eye? How could you have acquired an infection or an inflammation of the brain? Gosh, I hope whatever medication the Doctor gives you will help. Can't he be sure what caused the brain infection which paralyzed the nerve? When he says it's not serious, does he mean that it won't get any worse, or what?? The fact that he claims it can't be cured is enough to worry me. Why is he doubtful that nature will not cure it? Dearest, be sure and take your medication he gave you very regularly and faithfully. I guess you're getting new glasses, aren't you?? Be sure and let me know whatever develops. It always seemed to me that by your reactions the glasses you wore were too strong or the correction was too great. Take very good care of that left eye, Honey Bunch.

Dearest, I'm going to send home $30 by money order. Now I don't want you to save the money. In the first place, I owe you $50 from way back and so many other things that you'll have to pay for. Say, what's this you're telling me about owing $31.12 more on my 1943 income tax! Heavens alive, I paid that way back in March of last year. I paid -just a minute I just remembered now what that's for. I withheld 1/2 of the previous year's tax which was $62.25 and paid only 1/2 of that so I owe $31.12. Well, Hon, you can use this $30 to pay it or let it go till I come home.

[Friday] February 9th

Gee, we're having some of that snow you people had a few weeks ago. It's snowing fast and it's very dark outside. This is the first day of its kind for a few weeks. You tell that Ouija Board it doesn't know what it's talking about when it says we're waiting until 1949, that's at least three years late. How about it?

That's very interesting having a customer from Switzerland and her brother is from Italy. That place she was telling you about I saw a little, but I'm not at all near there now.

[Saturday] February 10th

I think you'd better not get my driver's license. If and when I get back this year, we can easily run up to Harrisburg in a half-day and get them personally. I'd gladly drive to Harrisburg without my license. Ha! Ha! For that matter, you can drive me up. How about it, Honey Bunch???

My Dear, would you or your parents mind too much if you'd send me Howard's address?? I don't know if I could find out anything but I think maybe I could if I'd know his address. I feel sure I could at least find out a few things. Have you heard anything more regarding him?

Do you mean to tell me, Honey Bunch, that you got stiff shoveling snow?? My oh my, did I laugh when I read that letter. Yes, you must be getting old. Of course, I guess there was a lot of snow too. Ha! Ha!

Say, Honey, if you happen to come across any fruit juice in cans you can send me some. I believe that'll taste very good. Potato chips and nuts would taste pretty good too if you get time to send them.

Before I started this letter, I got my first haircut since Camp Swift. Gosh, did I look a mess. Of course, he didn't take any off the top as yet as that is still pretty short. The fellows think my hair is thicker since it's coming out. I'm not sure it's thicker but I'm sure it's not thinner and that's what counts. Ha! Ha! Gosh, these Italians certainly don't have the equipment to cut hair that we have. It took him about half an hour to cut my hair. He also shaved me. Guess what I paid him, two packages of cigarettes, a bar of candy, and a piece of gum. I usually trade my cigarettes for gum and candy but I saved a couple of packages to give the barber.

You know those three questions you asked the Ouija Board at Virginia Bowman's place, it answered quite right. In fact, they were all right about where I was at the time, where I was going, and what part of Italy I was going to. Isn't it strange that it hit it right??

[Sunday] February 11th

Gee Whiz, I haven't heard from my Dear in about five days. I can't in the world see where all the mail is.

Dear, that identification bracelet hasn't been off my wrist since I first put it on. Gosh, but you'll never know how much I like it!! It's the nicest gift you could have gotten me.

Honey, how is your eye?? Gosh, but I worry about that so much. You people should stay well like I am. Ha! Ha!

[Tuesday] February 13th

Yesterday I was unable to write any letter, I just didn't have the time or facilities to write. Sunday, I received eight letters in all. One was dated December 2nd and I received it on Feb. 11th. That had two trips across the Atlantic.

You tell me that the chain broke on your Locket!! My heavens, I can't see what was the matter with that chain. Where did you buy the other chain??

Yes, Ruth Dear, I understand perfectly how your parents must feel when matters concerning Howard keep coming up. It just brings everything to mind again. If, however, they want these insurance forms and forms with regards to his back pay filled out, I'd do so. Certainly, it doesn't do any harm. That won't keep him from coming back if he is alive and well and after all that is what counts.

No, I don't believe Mother and Grandma when they say they'd like to give you and Sister some Rook games. Personally, I believe both of you would like to beat the other team and I can't blame you one bit. How about it? Ha! Ha! You had better get in shape till I get home because I'll really be primed. Ha! Ha!

I certainly would have liked to see Richard also. I'd like to hear about his experiences. I'm sure he'd have quite a bit to tell us. He was in the South Pacific for over two years, wasn't he?? Does he and "Rocky" look well?? They are both such small fellows.

[Wednesday] February 14th

Today is Valentine's Day, my Dear. I'm afraid you will not have received my valentine I sent you as yet but it's on its way. I'm sorry I'm not able to get some of Pauline's candy for all of us to enjoy but there will be other years.

My Dear, how is your eye?? Maybe you should see some eye specialists in New York or Philadelphia? Maybe they could cure the condition for you. Take the best care, please.

Say I never received that letter in which you told me where your Father had the accident? Did he receive that piece of chromium that was cut out from the light reflector?? I'm very glad that he likes the seat covers so much. That was as fine a gift as we could have gotten.

[Thursday] February 15th

This is the first letter I've written at night for some time. It's not easy to write by candlelight and that's all we have here in Italy. What a difference when I get back to "civilization" and electric lights again. Gosh, there are so many little things that a fellow misses that he'll really appreciate when he returns.

Gosh, remember all those newsreels we used to see showing how muddy it was in Italy, how vehicles and equipment were so hard to move because of it. Well, we're experiencing plenty of mud right now. It's just about "knee-deep" at some places and that's not exaggerated either.

My Dear, you asked about my watch in one of your letters. She's still operating okay but I'm expecting trouble any day. The first few days I've been over here I broke the crystal. I recovered part of it, put it back in place, and put adhesive tape over the rest of the face. It's holding pretty well but I can't expect too good results from such a "contraption". I have no idea where I can get another crystal.

You asked me, my Dear, how often I shave? Well, that varies. I try to shave about every two days and I don't miss too often. By gosh, it seems the less you shave the slower the whiskers grow. Speaking of baths, I had my first real bath yesterday. We were taken to a town where we took "showers" and were given all clean clothes. Gosh, I felt like a new man. Clean from head to foot for the first time in many a day.

Oh, by the way, I was told that I got a P.F.C. rating. You know, you kidded me about not earning enough money for us. Well, my stock evidently went up by $4.80 a month. Do you love me more now, my Dear?? Ha! Ha! Ha!

[Friday] February 16th

Honey Bunch, late last night I received a V-Mail letter from my Dearest mailed Feb. 2nd. Yes, it looks like V-mail travels faster than airmail but you can't write enough. I enjoy your long letters so much my Darling.

[Saturday] February 17th

Last night I received "9" letters. I read letters for two hours last evening without stopping. Thanks also for sending those articles from the papers concerning the various sports events? You know how I enjoy them. As a rule, our food is quite good. We've gotten canned rations rather frequently but not nearly as much as I thought we'd get. Don't worry your hubby still has plenty of flesh on his bones.

Where are you going on your vacation this year?? You must go somewhere and do something, Honey. Say, I'm so anxious to see how those new glasses are going to fit you. I certainly hope your eye will get better. Be sure and let me know how things are.

Say, Hershey doesn't seem to be doing so very well in the leagues. By the standing you sent me they were six points behind Buffalo and now I believe they're even farther behind. Boy, will we see the Hockey Games when I return.

[Friday] February 23rd

Six days have gone by since I was last able to write. I hope you won't worry too much about me not writing. I guess you can probably guess why I haven't written. Honestly, I haven't had a single opportunity to write. I'm writing this letter under rather unfavorable conditions and I'm hoping and praying that it will be mailed rather quickly. I shall relate more of my experiences and try and answer all your questions when I have more time. Please, My Dear, keep writing even if you fail to hear from me. I'm very well and everything is O.K. here.

[Saturday] February 24th

You can probably guess what I've been doing. I'm getting a "breather" today so I'm taking the opportunity to write home. My Darling, I've already told you that I'm part of the 10th Division and we are part of Mack Clark's[58] 5th Army.

Honey Bunch, one of the letters I got last night was mailed on Feb 15th and I received it on the 23rd. Eight days for an Air Mail letter. Gosh, that was a wonderful time, wasn't it?? My paper is in pretty bad shape, but it's all I have so I'm afraid it will have to do. I'm writing this letter right out in the open air. Honey, I've often heard about how valuable a fox hole can be, and believe me I was never so glad for one as I was the last few nights. I've built myself a "home" in Italy. Ha! Ha! Ha!

Dearest, I'm sorry to hear that you didn't feel well on the weekend of the 6th (Jan). Yes, Honey, that first communion I guess was pretty hard but we must realize how uncertain life is and just take everything that comes. Let's never lose our faith or our courage. I'm sure He'll watch over us all. I'm glad to hear that your parents are taking things so very well. Encourage them and brighten their day. You're such a good "trooper", my Dearest. Glad to hear that you had a good meal

---

[58] Mack Clark was the youngest 3 Star General in the US during World War II. He commanded the 5th Army in the Italian Campaign and accepted the German surrendered in Italy in May 1945.

up home. Those "dishes" you mention make my mouth water, especially the banana pie.

In one of your letters, you ask about my complexion!! Honey, I don't know right now how I look!! I haven't shaved for over a week and I haven't looked in a mirror for that time either so I presume I look a mess. I haven't even washed my hands in about five days but I'm well and healthy.

My heavens, what a dream you had about me being the Doctor's assistant!! What did you eat before you went to bed that night?? Ha! Ha!

Yes, the Ouija Board must have really lied if it said I was going to "Greece". It mustn't have known how to spell Italy. Mother and Grandma, I believe, really do have faith in it.

Honey Darling, things are moving rather fast right now in Italy and I'm never sure when I'll be able to write so please don't worry if you fail to hear for some time. Rending 1st Echelon Medical Service keeps a fellow rather busy when his troops engage in combat.

[Sunday] February 25th

I guess you're just about getting ready to go to Sunday School by now. Well, I wish I could be enjoying the Sunday with you but instead, I'm over in Italy doing what little I can to get this war over. Honey, I'm writing this letter sitting in my "foxhole". It seems a bit safer here than anywhere else and I can actually say I wrote a letter in a foxhole. Ha! I don't know if the chaplain will be able to have services where we are but I've already read the "Scriptures" so I've observed the Sabbath at least in part.

Ruth Darling, you've asked so frequently about my meals. Well right now, for the last week I've eaten nothing but "C" and "A" rations. You think at first you can't stand them but in time you get used to them. If you have time to build a fire and heat them, they're not bad at all.

My Dearest, you seem so very much annoyed by your new glasses. Gosh, I hope they'll work out alright. Please don't think about that line that runs across. You're probably thinking about that more than necessary. Give yourself plenty of time to get used to them. Now be sure and take your medicine. You still know who's boss? Ha!

Did your parents fill out that form concerning Howard's "back pay"? You said you had taken it into the Red Cross to have them explain it!! Yes, I presume many details have to be straightened out when such unfortunate incidences arise. As I said before, we must still maintain hope despite what seems to be a so-called closed case. There are always those instances where the War Dept. is wrong. Let's pray they are in our case.

Honey Darling, I've told you many times that I'm rendering 1st Echelon Medical Services. That includes first aid on the "field" and the transportation of wounded to their First Aid Station. Yes, I would very much like to meet up with Dr. Matthews. Mother sent me his address. If I ever get around to it, I might drop him a line.

I'm beginning to believe that you and Sister are becoming a lot more generous in giving some Rook games to Grandma and Mother. How about it?

Darling, I'm quite amused in hearing you buying a dog. Gosh, did I laugh when I read the letter. Of course, it's perfectly all right with me for you to buy a dog. I don't know, however, if I'd pay $25.00 for one but I'm sure she must be real cute, and if you enjoy having her why that's perfectly all right with me. If at all possible, take a picture of her and send it to me. Always glad to have another picture of my Honey. You ask me if I miss you and love you as much as ever??

Holy Smokes, I wish you knew how much I missed you and loved you. You'll never know but just you wait until I get back. Then you'll really find out. Ha! Ha! Ha!

I've never gotten the letter where you say you saw that Humphrey Bogart picture "To Have and Have Not". You mentioned in a few that you'd probably go. Gosh, I certainly hope you did. As I've said before you don't get enough entertainment.

[Monday] February 26th

I'm writing this letter in my foxhole as I did the one yesterday. Practically all the fellows around me hit water in theirs. I was fortunate enough not to have hit water. Sleeping in a wet and damp hole is not pleasant, believe me. I sleep fairly well in mine when you get a chance to sleep. I was in mine for about four hours last night. [the next line and a 1/2 had been cut out]

Last night I hit the jackpot again. I received 10 letters, well really only 8 and 2 Valentines. Once I get all my back letters, I can piece everything together. Gosh but I'm glad to receive your "real" kisses in your letters. You can't see my "real" kisses on my letters.

Let me mention again this "dog" incident. How come you changed your mind and bought a red "cocker" instead of a black one? Was it the fact that Aunt Marian had heard about this place in Douglasville? Red or black, doesn't make a particle of difference to me. Is this dog a pedigreed animal?? I think it should be for the price you paid.

Nine degrees below zero are pretty cold all right. Your Father must run into pretty much snow on his way to work. I guess by this time most of it has disappeared. You told me he took off his chains.

I have in front of me the letter you wrote on the 27th of January, the day you received my first letter. You went out with Sister for a "cocktail" consisting of banana ice cream. What a woman!! Ha! Ha!

Yesterday after I finished your letter, the chaplain did have services, and naturally, I attended. We sang familiar hymns and prayed several prayers. I felt much better after attending.

[Wednesday] February 28th

Have so much to write and so many letters to answer that I would very much like to write a longer letter but it's so late that a V-Mail will have to do. I received 8 letters today, four were from my Dear Wife and four were from the folks up home. They brighten my day so very, very much. Glad to hear you're starting to get my mail more regularly. I know just how you feel.

[Thursday] March 1st

The American Red Cross distributed some paper last night so I'm using it this morning. Well, I checked on all my letters this morning and I've gotten everyone up to and including Feb. 16th, isn't that fine!!

It's another beautiful day in Italy. Gosh, but we can be thankful that for the past two weeks we've had clear weather. It made things much easier for us.

What was Mother thinking about when she called up at 10:00 in the evening?? She should know that my wife doesn't keep such late hours. Ha! Ha! You should be like your hubby. If there's no work for him he "hits" his hole at dusk already.

Yes, my Dear, I hope you go to church as often as possible. It seems you are missing church pretty much. Well, you better be prepared to go every Sunday when your "hubby" returns. Yes, I'm hoping that these future months will pass real rapidly but you must not despair. Just have plenty of faith and never lose your courage.

Don't expect too much hair on my head. I don't believe I've lost anymore but I certainly wouldn't call it extremely thick. Ha! Ha! My sinus condition seems rather well at the present. Let's hope it doesn't annoy me any further.

As I've mentioned before, I haven't even seen a pair of skis, much less worn a pair. The Army does funny things, you know. Yes, we must have at least three children, my Dear, if you want more, why we'll just have more. How's that??

Hon, $5 was a very nice gift for Sister's birthday. She wrote and said she appreciated the gift. Honey, the length of a day is just about the same here as it is back home. There is very little difference. You must not get angry at your manager so much. Just laugh off those things she does. I know what it means to take things like that.

My dearest, I never knew you sat on the sofa to write my letters. I always pictured you as writing at the desk. Well, I know now exactly where you are practically the whole day.

Tell your parents that I'm constantly thinking of them and my good wishes go out with every letter I write to you. I understand why writing would be rather difficult.

[Friday] March 2nd

Yesterday I received another letter from my Dearest and also two letters from Mother which contained only newspapers, one the sports section of the Times and the other the "funnies" from one Sunday.

Yes, my Dear, I know what letters can mean to a person. That's the only thing that keeps a fellow going over here. Receiving mail just "peps" a guy up and he can take practically anything.

Honey, that letter you received from that officer concerning Howard sounds mighty interesting. Gosh, I would very much like to check up on that latter statement he made concerning the place where Howard is "supposedly" buried. Ruth Dearest, right now I'm in the Northern part of Italy but if I ever get the opportunity I'm going to look into the matter. As you said, I certainly think too that they would have known that much earlier and let us know then. Don't have too much faith in what he said.

Yes, my Honey, I can hardly get over the fact that Sister went to church with you on the 28th of Jan. What in the world is happening to her?? Is she getting religious all of a sudden?? Well, that was mighty nice of her anyway, don't you think?

What in the world is happening to you, falling all over the city streets?? Ha! Ha! It seems as though when such things happen in a day it happens two or three times. Did you receive any "open" cuts or bruises?? Please, my Darling, be more careful and take care of yourself. You know there's only one "you" and by gosh I don't want anything to happen to you.

Honey, I would take the meals we got back in the states anytime over these, but I'm getting along fine on what I'm eating. It provokes me sometimes the way fellows are always "grinding" and "complaining" about something.

My Dearest, if I were you, I'd ask them at the Internal Revenue Office what to do about my Income Tax. They'll be able to give you the best advice.

Every night I plan on something else which we must be sure and do upon my return. We'll have much to look forward to.

[Friday] March 2nd

Ruth Dearest, I'm writing a second letter in one day. I'm quite sure I won't be able to write tomorrow so I thought I'd get it written tonight. Today is Friday and we had church services, believe it or not. I presume we won't be having services on Sunday because everyone will be pretty busy.

Guess what, today I met a Lt. who went to Franklin & Marshall College. He graduated in 1942 and he remembers those football games on Thanksgiving Day when we always played them. I met another fellow from Reading by the name of Dixon. I found out he drove a "streetcar" for the Reading Transit Company. He drove car No. 71 on the Riverside-Cotton Street run. If I would have had more time, I could have talked to him for hours.

[Monday] March 5th

We are on the move again and I just didn't have an opportunity to write. Gosh, but it's cold today. I can hardly write my hands are so cold. For the last two nights, I've slept in an old building on some straw. Gosh, but it's a lot better than in a foxhole anyway. I hope this letter will get off pretty soon, but I can't be sure when I can mail it. I haven't as much as seen any skis and as for mountain climbing, we got that alright when we came into combat. We got "it" under fire!!! Ha! Ha!

Honey, how are your new glasses coming?? Gosh, you didn't mention anything about your eye or your glasses for quite a few letters. Does the glare of the sun still affect you, or is it better?

Didn't you buy any shoes yet, my Darling?? Gosh, you must be walking on your stocking feet the way you're complaining of not having any shoes. Ha! Ha!

As I've said in many of my previous letters, I'm in the Northern part of Italy and I'm a part of the 10th Mountain Division which in turn is a part of the 5th Army. We're on the front lines for the last two weeks, at least.

My dearest, I'm a very good boy!! You can trust me to the "tee". Gosh, what girls I've seen don't touch the fingernail of your small finger.

[Tuesday] March 6th (1 PM)

I presume my Dearest you are just about finished with your breakfast by this time!! How close have I come??? You know, I can see you going through your whole day from the time you get up in the morning until you retire at night, even though I'm 5 hours "ahead" of you.

You people are constantly asking me for requests. So, I'll ask for some more. It seems that toothpaste is rather scarce, so you can enclose some of that. Nestles' cocoa you mentioned in one of your letters would be fine; also candy, pretzels, and potato chips. I didn't receive any boxes at all but we were told there are quite a few at the post office and we'll get them when we're pulled back for rest.

Yes, Ruth, I'll tease Mother about putting salt in the sugar bowl. My, oh my, I bet you people teased the life out of her. Gosh, I bet that tasted horrible putting salt in your tea. Ha! Ha! Gosh, you had some more homemade ice cream. Say, put that on my list for every day for about two months, at least, when I get home.

[Wednesday] March 7th

I'm writing V-Mail today for I might be cut short. We might be on the move "again". Last night I didn't receive any mail so it's been two days now since I heard from my Wife.

My Dear, that boy who I treated who went to Father's school is in the infantry. I saw him about two weeks ago. He had been bitten by some sort of insect.

Gosh, but I'm glad you and Sister went to see Humphrey Bogart. I'm glad too that you enjoyed it. You must go to see more movies. Now that's an order. You still know who your "boss" is! Ha! Ha! Ha! No, I haven't seen any actors or actresses yet. I'm not particularly interested in them either. I see since Frank Sinatra was put in 4-F again he's going to tour Europe with a U.S.O. show.

[Thursday] March 8th

Boy, was I lucky this morning! I received six letters and three beautiful Easter greetings. Two letters were from up home and one from your good parents. Gosh, but that was nice of them to write to me. Glad to hear in today's letter that you received your income tax refund. If you don't need the money it would be swell to buy a War Bond. That indeed is a very good idea.

Honey, you don't have to worry about Sister "spoiling" our children. I'll have to tell her a thing or two. Ha! Ha!

[Saturday] March 10th

We were on the "move" again yesterday so I wasn't able to find an opportunity to write. Guess what was afforded us yesterday? I'm sure you'll never guess. Well, we were taken back for "showers" and then brought back to our holding positions. Gosh, was that something, to be able to wash in good hot water. We received clean O.D.'s, clean underwear, and socks. Of course, coming back, the dust was flying so badly that I presume I'm quite "filthy" again, but I was at least clean for a few minutes. Ha! Ha!

Say, my Dear, by this time you should have received my Valentine sent to you and also that $30 I remitted by money order. Gosh, you've never mentioned either. Please tell me as soon as you receive them.

Your bus really must have been late the night of the 8th of Feb. One hour and five minutes is a long wait. Do you wait outside of Whitner's until the bus comes in?? Gosh, but I certainly wouldn't!! You must go down to the waiting room.

You asked me about headaches, my Dear!! I've been fortunate. My headaches have been few and far between. Gosh, if I had all those headaches I used to have, I'd have a terrible time doing the things we're called upon to do. My feet are 100%. No trouble from them at all.

Yes, my Dear, I sleep quite well at night. No matter if I'm in a foxhole or if I'm on a cot like I did have for about 10 days in Feb. A fellow is really tired after a long day goes by.

What was John R. trying to do when he told those people about Howard's car?? I guess he figured he'd be able to get some sort of a "commission" out of it. I'm amused whenever I think of what he said to you concerning me not being able to stand the Army training. So, he thought I'd be getting my discharge!! Well, he certainly didn't call that one right. What have your parents decided to do about Howard's car anyway?? I can imagine how difficult that probably is. Of course, as you said in one of your letters, he'll probably want a newer car anyway when he gets back.

I'm glad you finally got some stockings. My Dear, you would have been walking around in your bare feet. Ha! Ha! In one of your letters, I received two days ago you asked about wearing "anklets" this summer. You wear just what you please. You mustn't ask me questions like that always.

Honey, the last two days we've been eating out of our mess kits. Dear, I haven't seen a table to eat on since we left the states.

[Monday] March 12th

For the first time since I've hit the shore of Italy, I'm feeling like a civilized human being. We've been pulled off the "front line" and are going to have a few days rest before we go back again. We're located in a fairly nice sized town, the name of which I undoubtedly cannot divulge at this time. I'm writing this letter at the Red Cross Service Club which is an extremely nice building, one of those old Italian aristocratic places.

They have a "GI" restaurant here and I ate there the last four meals. For the first time since I left the states, we ate off plates. You get a real good meal for $.10. You see the government runs it, I presume, and you get the full meal course for a dime. This noon I had macaroni, beans, and beef together with soup, bread, and jelly and dessert which was butterscotch pudding and a bun. This morning, I had oatmeal, two fried eggs, and bacon, and tomato juice. Gosh, it's like "Heaven".

Yesterday morning we got here just in time for me to make church services. I ran all over town looking for the place and here I found out for the first time in Italy I attended services where we had organ music and gosh, I felt good after attending. It seems that attending service relaxes a fellow so much. I have so much to be thankful for and gosh, I just had to give thanks.

This morning I looked up a jeweler in town but he doesn't have any watch crystals. He said I can get them in Florence, Rome, and Naples, however. It's amazing how well my watch works the way I have it patched up. Ha! Ha!

Yesterday I really was lucky. I received two boxes, the one from My Honey Bunch and one from Mother. Holy Smokes, was everything so very good and so welcomed.

Honey Bunch, please don't think I'm proud of myself for receiving that P.F.C. stripe. It couldn't have been too hard to receive or your hubby never would have gotten one. Ha! Ha! It seems the 10th Mt. Infantry Division has made a name for itself. Everyone over here is talking about the things they've done. Well, we'll be up there again before too long and Hitler's pup, Kesselring[59] better watch out. Ha! Ha! I see we've crossed the Rhine. Things might happen pretty fast now. Well, let's hope things will end in a hurry. I "wanna" get home and see my Honey. Does she still want me so badly? Maybe she's forgotten me? Ha!

Honey, you really must have had quite a time when you went to Douglasville for "Flush". Getting lost going and coming is somewhat of a record. Isn't It?? Ha! Ha! Ha! All kidding aside it must have been a mighty nice trip. I certainly wish I could see your dog "Flush". She really must be cute. Glad to hear that our car works so well. For about 65,000 miles the motor certainly runs smooth. I guess it must be the fellow who operated and took care of it. Ha! Ha! Ha!

The weather is lovely here. Naturally if anything it's warmer where we are now since we're more South.

Yes, I presume receiving the "Purple Heart"[60] made your parents feel bad. Of course, Ruth Dear, one must expect those

---

[59] Albert Kesselring was one of Nazi Germany's most skilled commanders who conducted the defense in Italy and was later tried for war crimes.

[60] This award was established by George Washington in 1782 and redesigned in 1931 being a gold rimmed heart with the image of George Washington in the center of a purple background, attached to a purple ribbon. In World War II it was awarded to those soldiers wounded or killed in action against an imposing enemy over and beyond the call of duty.

things. In time, it will be something that they'll be glad they have. Certainly, the government means well in sending it.

I appreciate, my Dear, that you keep impressing upon my Father that I'm alright. I know he constantly thinks I'm not well. Since he hasn't anything to occupy his mind he just sits and worries all the time. In practically every letter he writes to me he tells me what a good Wife I have.

[Tuesday] March 13th

Honey, guess what I saw 30 minutes ago? I was walking through town when I happened to glance to my right and there was an American-made automobile-a green 1937 Chrysler Coupe. I could tell it was Italian owned by the license. Gosh, was that something to see!

My Darling, I must thank you for sending all our folks Valentine greetings. Everyone has written and told me how pretty they all were. Yes, you must scold them for putting in a handkerchief in yours. Ha! Ha! It seems as though they are always one step ahead of us. Well, we'll get even with them somehow.

You asked about a PX? There aren't any PX's, my Dear, but within certain time limits, we receive some PX rations. They are bought right to your outfit. Right now, in the town we're in we live in rather large buildings. I believe the one I'm in had been some sort of hotel at one time.

Yes, I saw by the paper you sent that Abbot and Costello[61]played at the Astor!! Why didn't you go?? You always liked them so much. I can see where you're not listening to your "boss" so well. Ha! Ha!

---

[61] This was an American comedy duo that did stage, radio, movies and television during the 40's and 50's.

Say, according to the last standing of the Hockey League I saw Hershey better win a few games if they hope to make the playoffs. I presume the playoffs will start near the end of this month, won't they?? Gosh, I'm sure we'd go to some of the games if I were home. How about reserving some seats for us for next year's playoff?? Ha! Ha! Ha!

How's Flush and her "worms" by now?? I hope the medicine you got from Sam helped her.

[Thursday] March 15th

Gee, lately I'm just not able to write every day. I try as hard a possible but I just can't find the opportunity. Well, we're not in our nice town anymore. We've been moved "up" again.

Honey Darling, the night before last this fellow who's from New York who married a girl from Allentown asked me to go to a movie at the Red Cross Theater. Gosh, it seemed strange to see a movie. Ton Conway[62] was the leading actor. It was a murder story and I enjoyed it fairly well. It was so full when we got there I had to sit on the floor.

In your letter, you tell me about a new girl you got in your place. I can hardly get over the fact that she wants all her pay in War Bonds. I guess that's just about as patriotic a thing as anyone could do. My Dear, how much money do we have in War Bonds now that you've bought that $100 bond? You know they're in our safety box in the bank. If you want to ever get in to see them you just ask Mother for the key. I think she has it.

Honey, that's mighty fine denying yourself of something during Lent. I'm a bad boy for I haven't denied myself of anything in particular. Next year I hope to do better. As much

---

[62] He was a British actor known for playing private detectives.

as you like candy, I presume it's quite difficult to keep that denial.

You've asked me if most of the men attend worship services. I'm sorry to say that the percentage I think is pretty small. It seems though, that when the "sledding" gets pretty tough there are more people at services.

Well, Dear, you've fixed all our income taxes for '43 and '44. I guess that's the best. So, the government owes us $.33 for 1944. Gosh, but that's a large sum of money. Ha! Ha!

You know what Honey, you cheat at Rook, I believe. Ha! Ha! Gosh, must I laugh when I read how you and Sister talk across the table. I bet that makes Mother and Grandma mad doesn't it??

Wasn't that a coincidence?? Your Father finding that chromium strip the day he bought another one, and trying so hard before that to find it. Gosh, that's the way things always go.

[Friday] March 16th

Well, we've moved "up further" again and we really are there now!

Gosh, will I enjoy those Hershey Almond bars, 48 bars in all! Man, you'll spoil me sending all that good candy. Thanks so much for them.

Ruth Dear, did you receive your Beautician License by this time? You know last year it took such a long time to receive that license. I can't in the world see what makes that Bureau of Professional Licensing so very slow.

Honey Darling, about the questions you asked me in your letter of the 29th I can say that I'm doing all three of those things. You see when you get into combat and things start "popping", you do everything. They need you all over the place.

Yes, My Dear, I'll scold Sister for telling you she's going to push you out of bed. Ha! Ha! I guess she never did push you out of bed, though did she?? Were you and she fighting since she said something like that?? If that keeps up, I'll have to come home and settle you two. I guess you're laughing now, aren't you? Ha! Ha!

Say, it's a wonder Mother wouldn't put your letters from me out on the "doorstep" so that you'd see them more quickly than if they'd be on the coffee table. Just kidding my Dear!! That's indeed a very good idea. I can just imagine how much you enjoy receiving mail for I know how good I feel upon getting some.

Yes, my Dear, I'm still carrying your pictures with me and they'll always be with me. Gosh, but I don't know what I'd do without your pictures. I just love to look at you.

[Saturday] March 17th

Gosh, my Dear, I'm writing on whatever paper I have available and I'm sure it won't matter to my Dearest. I haven't got all my belongings with me and at the moment I grab paper whenever I possibly can. Today it's another beautiful clear day. Last night it cleared and there were lots of stars in the sky. Gosh, we can be very fortunate if we don't get any rain this spring because it gets muddy in Italy when it rains.

Well, I presume you're starting another busy Saturday back home. Over here a Saturday is no different than any other day in the week. How is that strike coming back home? By gosh, those fellows are starting to disgust me. They can gladly come over here and fight. I'll come back home and run the buses and trolleys and won't kick about my wages either. Ha!

My Dearest, we eat our meals whenever we get an opportunity, but usually, at the times we've been used to eating. In the C rations, the desert can have either coffee, lemon juice, orange juice, or cocoa. I usually exchange my coffee packet for any of the others or else if I do get coffee, I just don't drink anything. I don't believe that the Army will ever get me to like coffee.

Honey, you should never ask me if I love you yet because if you knew just how much I do love you I believe you'd faint. You'll never know how fortunate I consider myself in having such a good and faithful wife. I sent my Dearest an Italian Easter Greeting. I certainly hope she receives it by Easter. Easter comes this year on "April Fool's Day", isn't that a coincidence??

Honey, the men we treat are men who are wounded in action. Understand??? The answers to your first and second questions of 2/23 are both yes. Honey Bunch, I travel right with the combat unit, understand??

Glad that you found a girl that doesn't smoke or drink. Boy, that's something rather scarce, those girls are few and far between. She really must be quite a nice girl.

So, Franklin and Rachael are expecting a baby. Well, they're indeed mighty lucky but I am sure not any luckier than we are and will be in the future.

[Sunday] March 18th

Has spring arrived as yet? You mentioned in one of your letters that the days are getting noticeably longer. Gosh, that's what I like about spring and summer, those long nights when you can be out in the yard or take a drive with the car. Gosh, but there are so many things that I'm planning on when I return that it will take us a while to catch up. Ha! Ha!

Say, my Dear, aren't you driving the car yet this spring?? Heavens, the snow is gone by now so I should think you surely would have taken the Chevy out. You don't have to rely on your Father to take you up home anymore. Here's another thing, the present group of gasoline coupons run out on the 22nd of the month. Be sure you make use of ours.

Honey, about that question you asked in your letter of 2/22 as to setting up temporary hospitals after each town is taken, that isn't quite what is done. When we advance, the Battalion Aid Station moves up also and is usually about 300 yds. to the rear of the combat units. To this station, wounded men are first evacuated. Of course, it depends on the type of operation and the terrain just where that Aid Station will be set up.

Dearest, there won't be any training in mountain climbing either. All the mountain climbing we get is that in actual combat and we've experienced quite a bit of that. Ha! Ha! Ha!

I see that on the 22nd you and Sister were very good to Mother and Grandma in giving them two out of three Rook games you played. I wonder sometimes about your giving them the games. Ha! Ha! I believe that all four of you try desperately hard to win the games. I don't know if I'll play with you or not when I get back if you cheat so much and talk across the table. I won't know how to act because you know I don't in the least know how to cheat. Ha! Ha! I'm so glad that Sister likes to play.

So, you dreamt I was at Camp Abilene, Texas?? You got the city and camp mixed up a bit. Yes, that was a mighty nice dream alright. We did have a real nice time those four weeks you were at Abilene.

Thank you for sending me Howard's address. I'll see what I can find out. I already know that he was in the 157th Infantry Regiment which was part of the 45th Division. The 45th Division is now fighting in the Western Front. As to "Matterhorn", I know where it is but I'm not there, "as yet".

[Tuesday] March 20th

Last night I was up most of the night. Up until about 1 AM I stood guard on the phone line in case they'd call for a Medic. At about 4 AM we treated a half dozen men who had been wounded. For the last three nights, I've been quite busy.

I'm still the same fellow you saw on November 29th. Gosh, I can still see you on the platform at the "Outer Station". It was raining and rather nasty that night wasn't it?? Gosh, the train was late so we had a few extra minutes together, didn't we???

Both you and Sister have gotten the wrong slant on what was going on the 4th of February. Don't worry, we did not retreat!! Instead, we engineered our first big attack if you could call it that, however, it wasn't anything compared to what we did starting the 20th of February. Dearest, you are exactly right about the 10th Division and the 85th Infantry taking part in the battle of Mt. Belvedere.[63] I was definitely in that battle.

[Wednesday] March 21st

I've seen in the Stars and Stripes that we got yesterday that the U.S. is enjoying rising temperatures in the last few days. Harrisburg had 83 degrees last Saturday and Mission, Texas had 95 degrees. This morning I got mail for the first time in three days.

Gosh, but I'm sorry that some portion of my letter on the 26th was cut out. Please don't be inquisitive about it. It probably wasn't much. I'll try and not write anything that will

---

[63] This mountain is the highest in the Apennines Mountain Range in Northern Italy. The Germans had taken a stronghold there for nearly six months. On February 18th the 10th Division started a night assent over ice and snow to take Riva Ridge and then continue to take the mountain. This ended victorious but with a loss of nearly 1,000 American soldiers.

be cut out and yet I know you're wondering where I am and what I'm doing, so I might be getting a bit "careless" lately.

Yes, my Sweet, by 1949 there'll be two or my name isn't Snyder. Ha! Ha! Aren't you willing?? You know I must keep alive the name Snyder. Ha! Ha! Say that dog Flush really must be requiring a lot of attention. She's giving your Mother quite a time.

[Thursday] March 22nd

Thanks a million for sending that picture of you and Barry. Gosh, Dear, but that was a good picture. My honey is just too beautiful for words and I see she has the locket on. I showed the picture to some fellow soldiers and guess what they said? "How did a good-looking woman like that ever fall for a guy like you"?

[Friday] March 23rd

Well according to your letter of the 11th you're going to bring our bedroom suite to your place. Well, that's perfectly alright with me. Are you still as crazy about it as you were when we bought it? I hope it's still in its "new" condition. Have they "skinned" it any by leaving it on display?? Just what did we pay for it, anyway? Was it some $200 or $300 or was it even more??

`Honey Bun, you're a very bad girl!! You must go along to the movies with Sister or anyone else for that matter, who invites you. I've told you that time and time again. Here she wanted you to go along a few weeks ago and you didn't. Are you that anxious to get my mail?? Ha! Ha!

My Darling, all the decisions you are making in my absence are quite sound and logical. I'm real proud of my wife. Honey Dearest, you're spending entirely too much money on food for me and boxes and the like. I'll just have to stop asking for requests if you spend so much. I guess you know how much I like cashew nuts but were they $3.25 a pound? That's entirely too much to pay for nuts.

That really must be a nice "log"[64] that your parents bought from the money you gave them for their Anniversary. That must be very lovely when that revolving light is on. Yes, we'll have to make "love" in that romantic atmosphere. How about it? You like to think of those things, don't you??

[Saturday] March 24th

Well, I've seen in the Stars and Stripes that Hershey beat Indianapolis in the first game of the semi-final series. Buffalo also beat Cleveland in their first game. I would have liked to have been home to see some of those games.

Today this morning I believe I've had the worst headache I've had since in the Army. I thought my head would split. Every time I'd move my head it would "pound" something awful. I took two aspirin and now it feels much better. I stood guard on the phone last night from 8 to midnight and I felt it coming on when I went to bed.

I still haven't seen Ed. I have no idea when I'll see him again either. We'll certainly have a lot to talk over if we'd get together again.

We'll take all the walks you want to when I return. I too will enjoy them I guess a lot better than these hikes and marches one takes in the Army. Ha! Ha!

What do you mean by saying you're not going anywhere on your vacation?? I'm ordering you to go somewhere, at least to several movies. That's an order. Gee, remember last year we both were having our vacation at the same time, everything was planned and here Uncle Sam grabbed me.

---

[64] I believe this must have been some sort of "fake" fireplace item, where the revolving light made it look like a burning fireplace.

Gosh, did I "wiggle" that right week at work, and the next week I received my induction notice. Well, that's the way life is!

You received an Air Mail letter in eight days. Boy, that was a wonderful time. Just a little over a week. Isn't it funny, the letter I write the next day might take two weeks or longer.

No Darling, a fellow stays in his foxhole day and night. It's his "home". Ha! Ha! Yes, some fellows dig two and three-man holes. I usually dig alone. The last one I dug with another fellow, boy, was he "nervous in the service". Ha! Ha! Aren't we all?? Naturally, things aren't as pleasant as they can be but this is war and I hope that it'll soon be over.

[Sunday] March 25th

Today is Palm Sunday!! Yes, I certainly would like to be home over this coming week. Easter's a great day in the church, isn't it? I guess your other boyfriend will have to buy you your corsage this year because I can't find any over here in Italy that would be good enough for my Darling Wife. Ha! Ha! I've been trying all day to find out when and where church will be held but nobody seems to know. If I don't manage to get there, I'll conduct my own services. Never have I thought about Palm Sunday and its significance more so than I have this year.

Say, Honey Bunch, by the 1st of April you'll have to get new license plates for the Chevy. I guess they only cost $10 again this year. Have you had any trouble with the tires? Has that other new inner tube on the front wheel given you any trouble? I just bought those front tires a short time before I was inducted. This was the year we had planned to buy a new car. I figured I'd trade our present one but the way things look we'll hang on to it for a while. Gosh, I'm anxious to see what those new cars are going to look like. That's another "hobby" of mine.

Yes, the war news looks very good at the moment. Let's hope it continues and the victory will be ours in the very, very near future. We seem to be progressing very well on all fronts. I guess you know by this time that the commander of German Forces in Italy, Field Marshall Kesselring has been named Commander of the German Forces on the Western Front. Let's hope that will lower the morale of the German soldier in Italy.

Glad to hear you wrote to Francis. You know he wrote to me and I answered him. He addressed his letter "somewhere in France". Since then, he has moved to Belgium and probably by now is inside Germany. I'm sure he'll be very glad to hear from you.

So, films are rather scarce in Reading?? Yes, I'd like a picture of Flush but I'd rather have some more pictures of you and don't say you're horrible looking either. My Honey is very, very beautiful and I'm not the only one who says that.

Yes, I well remember how scared my Dearest is of thunder and lightning!! You mustn't be afraid of those things. So, you were wishing you could "cuddle" up close to me and I would protect you. What will you do this summer when you'll get lots of storms?? I'm afraid you'll find someone else to protect you!

[Wednesday] March 28th

Well, my Dearest, we've moved again and I'm rather tired. We walked a goodly portion of the night and gosh, the weather is miserable. It's the type of weather which one always associated with Italy. It's raining and boy does it get muddy in a hurry when it rains.

Today I hit the jackpot as far as mail goes. I received nine letters, wasn't that just fine? One of them was from "Ed". Gosh, but I was glad to hear from him. He said I should thank you from him for that fine Easter greeting you sent him.

[Thursday] March 29th

Gosh, things happen quickly!! Today I was told that I was going on pass tomorrow to Florence.[65] They say it's a good break. I was one of the first fellows from our Medical Section to have the opportunity. I don't know as of yet how long I'll be able to stay but even for few days will be O.K. I was told that those men who had worked hardest and accomplished the most were the first to receive passes. I don't know what there is doing in Florence but I'm told you get a "cot" with a mattress on it and I'm sure I'll get my "twelve" hours of sleep and probably more so. Honey Darling, you can feel safe for the next few days.

[Friday] March 30th

Well, my Honey, I received my pass and I'm spending four or more days in Rest Camp in one of the largest cities in Italy. No one else is with me from my own Medical Section but I like to be alone. I can do just as I please without taking orders from anyone. The only thing I won't like about this rest is that I won't receive any mail till I get back and gosh, I can hardly wait to receive my mail.

From what little I've seen of the city it's quite nice, but give me Reading any day. I'll be able to celebrate Easter here and on Saturday at 11 AM there will be services here in the

---

[65] Florence was occupied by the Germans from 1943 to 1944. In May 1945 the US Army's Information and Educational Branch started an overseas university. Several thousand students would pass through its 4-month course.

Red Cross building which is a part of the building where I sleep.

[Saturday] March 31st

Well, I've spent my first full day here at my rest camp. You can forget the war and act like a human being again. Ha! Ha! The mail clerk said before I left that he'd have to hire a "mule" to carry all the mail I receive. Yes, I believe, I receive more mail than anyone else in our Medical Section. Of course, I write more also at least that's what the Lt.'s say who censor our mail.

We eat in a dining room similar to the one we ate at in the other city, but here you don't pay a single penny. This noon for dessert I had ice cream and cake. This morning I got up about 7:30 and had breakfast which consisted of wheat cereal, bacon & eggs, bread and jelly, and good water. Water you know, is sometimes hard to get. Usually, one must purify his own before he can drink it. [66] Then I went down in the basement and took a good hot shower and got all clean clothing.

Dearest, I hope you won't get mad at me but they have a place here in the building where they take your picture and I decided to get a few taken. Of course, I got a shave right here also (it cost 5 cents. Ha! Ha!). I'm doubtful the pictures will be very good. He snaps you before you know it and I'm sure I must have been in a very awkward position. If they don't get very good, I'll just tear them up.

After that, I came into the Red Cross and read the Stars and Stripes. They have real comfortable chairs. It took me until noon till I finished the paper. In fact, I guess I "dozed"

---

[66] Halzone tablets (made from chlorine compound) was supplied with a soldier's C rations. Two tablets could disinfect a quart of water. The water would end up smelling and tasting of chlorine but was safe to drink.

off a few times. You know I'm not used to having such comfort. Ha! Ha! Believe me, I never thought Luke Snyder would ever have the "guts" enough to undertake and experience what I did and I guess maybe the "higher-ups" appreciate it.

I bet that must have been a riot seeing Flush climb the front stairs taking that runny. I understand exactly what you mean. She seems to be requiring a lot of care lately. Say, I didn't know the "picture album" or whatever you call it that Sister gave you was small enough to carry in your purse. Heavens, you mustn't look at those pictures so much, or soon you'll begin to get tired of that husband of yours.

This afternoon I just walked and walked viewing the more important places of the city. These Italians are devout Catholics and gosh there are beautiful cathedrals here. Every carving and painting has a definite significance. This place must have had an elaborate transportation system, almost every street has tracks on it, but of course, no more trolleys are running. The Italian automobiles are peculiar-looking little things. They are much smaller than our cars.

Gosh but I'm glad that my Dearest has started to drive the car again. You tell me you enjoy driving and I'm glad to hear that. I guess by the time I get home you won't even let me drive anymore. Ha! Ha!

Honey Bunch, Major General Hays[67] is the Commanding Officer of the 10th Division and Colonel Barlow commands the 85th Inf. Understand??? Gosh, you're sure acquainting yourself with the 10th Division activities, aren't you?? I wonder why?? Ha! Ha!

---

[67] He took over in 1944 and arrived in Italy with his troops in January 1945. At the end of the war, he became High Commissioner for the US Occupation Zone in Germany from 1949

Dearest, no matter how dirty a fellow's hands are he can apply bandages and the like, they are absolutely sterile, have no fear!! And then too, sulfa powder and pills[68] take care of any infection, so why worry.

[Sunday] April 1st

Well, Easter of 1945 has rolled around and it doesn't seem right that I'm not there to celebrate this great day with My Honey Bunch. Well, I certainly hope that my Dear Wife will have a very happy and pleasant Easter and that when Easter rolls around in 1946, we'll be spending it together. Would that suit my Wife, O.K.?

They had a very nice Easter service. They had a choir and one of those portable organs. We even had the Army and Navy hymn books.

Honey, you mentioned again about sending an impression of my watch crystal. Well, I forgot to tell you I've left my watch with a jeweler here and I'll be able to get it before I go back to the "line". He'll put a crystal in for $7.50, a little more than we'd pay in the states but that's O.K. By the way, in the Stars and Stripes today I saw that tomorrow morning at 2 o'clock we turn our watches ahead an hour. It's called "B" time or British Summer Time. It will go back again probably in September.

I look forward to a Sunday when I can attend worship services. This really should be a very encouraging Easter because Peace I believe is not too far distant. Let's only hope and pray that nothing will happen to us until we're able to be together again.

---

[68] Sulfa powder was thought to have an important affect on preventing infection but it was later confirmed that debridement and secondary closure of wounds was most efficient for healing.

Gosh, but my Honey is becoming "brave". Ha! Ha! Once she backs the car out of the garage all by herself, she is really quite good. And you went over to the drugstore for the papers too. I always knew my Honey Bunch was a very good driver. I guess she takes after her husband. Ha! Ha!

I must laugh when I think of the time you had with Flush. She wouldn't move at all as long as she was on the leash but as soon as you took it off, she'd come along. Gosh, but she must be a cute dog. So, she knows her name already. You can't be mad at her for putting a hole in your stocking. She doesn't know any better.

[Monday] April 2nd

Well, this was my last full day on pass. Tomorrow morning I go back to my unit, at least I start back then. Gosh, I can hardly wait to go back so that I'll be able to receive my mail. Today I walked myself practically to "death" (Ha! Ha!) looking for some gifts. Honey, I bought you a few things and sent them already. 1) a pillowcase with the 10th Mt. Division insignia on it 2) a couple of handkerchiefs 3) a pair of earrings, if you want to wear them. Gosh, I didn't know what to get for my Folks. I finally saw a nice tea set with the 5th Army insignia on it. I bought that for all of them. You see, with the money I managed to have I couldn't buy what I would have liked to although what I did get should be good. If I ever get a pass again, I'll have to buy your parents something.

[Tuesday] April 3rd

Here I am again, my Dearest. We were scheduled to leave this rest area at 10:00 but I just found out that we won't leave until 1:00. Gee Whiz, I sure should have lots of mail when I get back to my unit, and believe me, I just can't wait to read it!! Say, I received those pictures I had taken. I received six of the "passport" size. They are so lousy looking I doubt very much whether I'll send them home. If you promise me you won't laugh or be too disappointed when you see them, I might consider sending them. Ha! Ha!

This morning I found a chap who wanted to play ping pong and I played about nine games. Gosh, did I sweat?? It's going to feel mighty strange to go back to our fox holes. Ha! Ha!

[Wednesday] April 4th

I'm back with my unit and while things here aren't like they are back in Florence, things aren't too bad. Last night I got back about 8:30 and there was the thing I'd been looking for the last five days, my mail. Guess how much mail I received?? I received seventeen letters, two boxes from my Wife and one from Sister. Holy Smokes I was up till after midnight reading letters by the light of a candle. In both boxes, there were some papers that I always enjoy reading. Also, in your letters, you had some interesting clippings. Say that really must have been some excitement in Reading when Tony Moran[69] was murdered. I didn't know him but I had heard plenty about him. He was connected with all the "underworld" movements and rackets. Did they catch the fellow "Wittig", his former pal who was suspected of his murder? There's too much happening at home, I must come back to take it all in!!

---

[69]Organized crime was very big in Reading during the 1920's through the 60's especially related to numbers, gambling and prostitution. Tony Moran was said to have been murdered by John Wittig in a shop on Penn Street. The motive was said to be revenge since Tony didn't help him get out of jail.

Gosh, I'm disappointed I didn't get my watch. It's still at the jeweler. I found a fellow who'll get it to me when it's finished and send it to me. I don't like the idea of sending it through the mail but it's the only way I know to get it.

One afternoon I had forgotten to tell you, I had gotten a bicycle for 3 1/2 hours and rode all over town. At the rest camp, they have 50 American-made bikes. It doesn't cost a single penny. I really think Uncle Sam takes good care of his men on passes. I was told that all passes and leaves have been canceled for the future. What that means I don't know, but I have a pretty fair idea.

[Thursday] April 5th

Last night I also received two more packages which made four in two days. Boy, you are keeping me supplied in everything! Gee Whiz, you mustn't send me any more juice. I see it cost 50 pts. and you sent all three cans. Heavens where did you get all those pts.? Yes, this morning I drank, with the help of another soldier, the third can so you can see how much we appreciate it. I really believe I have enough soap for the duration. Ha! Ha! Thanks very much for the National League Baseball schedule. I can follow the games now, even if I don't get the results the following day.

Dearest, you mentioned the "lot" opposite Grandpa's house, as to whether we should buy it or not. That's a very interesting problem. I hate to have him save it for us because it's hard to know exactly what one is going to do. It's wonderful of him to be willing to sell without requiring any immediate money. By the way, how much does he want to sell it for??

I don't know either what exactly "certain funds" could mean concerning Howard. I'm beginning to believe it might be some money or a valuable thing since they asked whether he had a "will" or whether he was married. Have you answered the letter or received any further information? I've passed by quite a few "American Cemeteries"[70] but I'm sure that if what that officer said concerning Howard is true, he'd be buried in a cemetery further south than one's I've seen. It's amazing to see how many of our "boys" have been buried "over here". Let's hope that a better world will emerge from this conflict and that they haven't died in vain.

Yes, the Red Cross had come right up to our foxholes that day. Yes, my Dear, we eat there too and at times one is very glad to eat there. Ha! Ha!

Yes, I understand how you felt when Mary told you Jack had to pay $67.00 out in tax money. I'd gladly pay that out if I'd be in his shoes. It seems people always gripe no matter how fortunate they are. It's the same way over here. We can be fortunate we're O.K., not hurt or killed and yet some men complain about "this and that". Some are never satisfied.

Dear, this morning I combed my hair and I believe a few hairs came out so I thought I had better tell you. Ha! Ha! Mother tells me that you aren't staying up home anymore because you don't like their beds now that you have our "suite" to sleep in. Is that right? Ha! Ha!

[Friday] April 6th

I'm writing V-Mail because we're going to be on the "move" again and you'll never know when you'll pull out. Yes Dear, both Sister and Mother like our bedroom suite very much. Well, I'm glad we bought a good one. I'm sure we'll be quite satisfied with it. I'll bet that "blue" spread sets it off nice.

---

[70] Florence American Cemetery Memorial covers 70 acres with head stones of over 4,000 U.S. Military. Included are those that fought in the Apennines shortly before the war's end.

[Saturday] April 7th

My Dearest Sugar Pie,

Well, how does my Wife like that name for a salutation?? Congratulations my Dear, on your increase in salary!! Gosh, but you're earning a goodly wage. However, if you ever need any money be sure and withdraw some from the bank. Never deprive yourself of anything you should have or would like to have.

The soldier who I had asked to get my watch returned to the outfit and he had gotten my watch. For the first time in over two months, my watch is in A1 shape. You know I've had this watch for eight years. My parents bought it for me when I graduated from high school.

Honey, don't tell me that you're afraid of a few "moths". Gosh, do I have to laugh! Really, my Dear, they won't hurt you. You should sleep with me some nights and enjoy my "bed partners". Ha! Ha! At the moment I'm staying in a building and straw is my bed.

Holy Smokes, do I have to laugh when I think of what you did before you went to bed that first night you slept in our new "bed". I mean putting my shoes under the bed. Gosh, but that was sweet, and if it made you feel better and sleep better why you just keep them there. So, you could just imagine me jumping in bed with you. Ha! Ha!

I read about your conversation with Norman's wife in the "shop" and knowing now what I know it just makes me feel bad. Why must such things happen!! And Norman was a fine fellow too and a very bright chap!! Sorry to hear about Donald being wounded again. Was he wounded badly or don't you know?

Dearest, don't you know gasoline is rationed!! What kind of driver are you, going all the way up to the "Center" school building to turn around? That's much worse than "stalling" a car at a hill!! You'd better not let the O.P.A.[71] find out!

[Sunday] April 8th

At 2 PM we had church service and I certainly am happy to be able to go. The last hymn we sang was that familiar communion hymn which I'm sure you too will be singing in a very few hours, "Just As I Am Without One Plea". Gosh, but that brought me home when we sang that hymn. The service was held beside a haystack.

I didn't receive any letters yesterday or today but I did get three packages and an envelope containing the newspaper clippings which told about "John Wittig" surrendering himself in connection with the "Tony Moran" murder. Gosh, but I enjoy reading about hometown news. Ha! Ha!

[Monday] April 9th

We always enjoyed Sunday so much. With the baseball season approaching, we would take in our share of ball games. Wouldn't we?? Now you must keep me informed as to how every team is making out. Tell Daddy that he too must keep in touch with what Southwest is doing. That will keep his mind on something.

Last night I received some mail and another package. Heavens, you people are "flooding" me with packages. I'm able to supply the whole Medical Section in food or rather "delicacies". I honestly believe nothing has been missing from any of the boxes so far.

Yes, Dear, I've met some nice fellows. Of course, the way things are, one doesn't get an opportunity to form too long an

---

[71] This was the Office of Price Administration whose responsibility was to limit who could purchase certain commodities like gasoline and set the quantities of rationed items citizens were allowed to buy.

acquaintance. Say, I don't know whether I liked what you said about me being a little "trying" when it comes to "streetcars". It's just a hobby of mine, that's all. Ha! Ha! Yes, Ed should have heard what this fellow had to say. I'm sure he'd have been quite interested.

I'm so glad that you had another good dinner over at the West Reading Hotel. What in the world was the matter with you girls when you took the wrong bus going to West Reading?? Heavens, all you had to do was take a West Lawn or Sinking Spring bus and get off right in front of the place. You people must have been blind! Ha! Ha!

As I told you before regarding that picture of us "kissing", you might get so anxious to "kiss" that you won't wait until I return. Be sure and let me know when you receive that package which I mailed in Florence. Maybe sometime later I'll be able to send you some more things.

[Tuesday] April 10th

Yes, My Dear, we've worn O.D.'s all the time since we left the states. However, for the last few weeks, we've been wearing what are known as "ski" pants or "mountain" pants. They really have the pockets in them (six in all). They seem a bit lighter in weight and lighter in color. Honey, we don't wear our blouses over here. When I was in Florence, they gave me what is known as an "Eisenhower blouse"[72] or an overseas blouse. I didn't like them as well as I did the blouse we wore on the "other side". My Dear, we only have "one outfit". We get clean clothing when we take showers and let the dirty ones there.

Say, my Dearest, you really must have been naughty dreaming the dreams you have been dreaming. You just

---

[72] This was coupled with a cropped jacket of wool which was knows as the "Ike" jacket since this was how he was usually dressed.

remember it and tell me all about it when I get back. Yes, we'll make up for a lot of things, won't we?? Do you know what I mean?? Ha! Ha!

What's My Sweetheart doing with all that money she's getting now??? Honestly, I'm proud of my Sweetheart. The company must know how good you are and realizes your assets. The "commission" you're getting during this Easter Season amounts to quite a bit.

$450 isn't too much to ask for Howard's car. With cars hard to get and processes what they are[73], that isn't too much.

I can hardly believe that people can be so narrow-minded as you say. I'm referring to people "snubbing" Aunt Kathryn because John is not overseas. No one can help with that. More power to him if he didn't have to come over. People aren't satisfied when you're in the service. They even want you overseas. In fact, if you're not "ten feet under" they think something's the matter. If people would only get over that jealousy and be friendly one to another.

[Wednesday] April 11th

Well, yesterday I received some more mail and it was quite a variety of mail at that. I received a letter from your Mother, from Sister, some funnies from Mother, an overseas edition of the Philadelphia Evening Bulletin (which was sent by my Uncle Alden), the Reading Newsweek from C. Steel, and a box of airmail stationery from my Darling.

---

[73] Car manufactures were converted into the war effort, making trucks, planes, tanks and cannon barrels. Cars were sold to those whose travel was critical to American life such as doctors, police, those working on the war effort and traveling salespersons. Chevy began producing cars again in the fall of 1946.

[Thursday] April 12th

I certainly didn't think I'd write today but things change quickly sometimes so here I am penning my usual letter. Say, my Dearest this is the third day I haven't heard from you!! Have you found another man and decided not to bother with your naughty "hubby" anymore?? Ha! Ha! Just kidding!! Your husband still is a great "teaser" as he's always been. I do wonder what is holding up your letters? I'm sure you are writing every day. I enjoy your letters so very, very much and I'm lost when I fail to hear from my Dearest Wife.

My Sweetheart, are you going to Washington on Monday to see the 1945 baseball season inaugurated? I'm sure you are!! Ha! Ha! Yes, I'm so anxious to see the coming baseball season open. Why don't you and your Father and Uncle Clarence, Jack and Mary go to see some games in Philadelphia? Then you'd have to tell me the whole story of the game from the first to the last pitch. Would you do that for me?

Poor Judy!! You say she's aging so lately. Gosh, but I'm sorry to hear that. She's such a nice dog and not knowing Flush as yet, she's the only dog I know well. When a dog reaches the age that Judy is you can't expect her to be so "peppy" anymore.

Has R. Kaufman left for the Navy already?? Two of Arlan's children will be in the Navy then. I'm glad that Frederick got a deferment. Gosh, if he'd have gone, they'd have all three sons in the service.

So, Francis is in the Infantry now?? No, I haven't heard from him since I last told you. At that time, he was still in the Quarter Masters Corps!! I hope to have an answer to the letter I wrote him. At that time, he was in France. I guess he's in Germany at this time.

Does Mother have a suntan this early in the year already?? She was so very "dark" last season. I'm so glad she likes to work in the yard. It does her worlds of good both physically and mentally. She never wanted me to see her in overalls. I must kid her about that when I write to her.

[Friday] April 13th
Today we're all saddened by the news of the death of our great President.[74] It seems as though it just can't be. He was our greatest friend. I only hope that it will not hinder the progress of the war or the peace negotiations that will follow. His death will make many of us see how wonderful an individual he really was. Gosh, but it will be hard on my Father. He admired him so much. You should be here to see the reaction when the news came. Well, we'll fight harder now than ever and we're going to win this war in a hurry and the peace that follows. If those conservative reactionaries cause any trouble, we'll have to defeat them at every turn.

[Wednesday] April 25th
I've run out of ink and we're traveling "light". I have plenty of ink but none with me. This will be a very short letter, just a few lines to let you know I'm O.K. Gosh, I hope you won't worry too much. The last letter I was able to write was on April 13th, I've been on the "go" ever since and I just

---

[74] History books show that in February President Roosevelt flew to Egypt and boarded the ship USS Quincy where he met with the King of Egypt and the Emperor of Ethiopia. He also held a historic meeting with the Founder of Saudi Arabia. He then met with prime Minister Winston Churchill and later with American Ambassadors to Britain, France and Italy. He returned to the US and addressed Congress on March 1st. He was described as looking "frail and sickly". On April 12th he died at the Little White House at Warm Springs, Georgia with what was diagnosed as a cerebral hemorrhage.

couldn't find the time or opportunity to write. Now when I'll be able to write again, I don't know but please don't worry. I received about 15 letters in the last 12 days. Hadn't received any in about five days but last night I got a "slew". I received three packages since I wrote you.

Lots of things have happened since I wrote. If you are following the papers you probably know what I mean. Once again, I can thank God many times for being able to write to my Dearest Wife. There are so many things that happened in the last 13 days that I would like to write but time will not permit. Later when things have settled down, I'll be able to relate more of my experiences.

Yes, it's just too bad about losing our great President!! He's a man we'll miss terribly. Those who fought against him will only now realize how great a man he is.

The weather has been very fine. It's hot during the day but the nights are quite chilly. It makes fox hole sleeping a little uncomfortable. Things happened so fast last April 14th that I lost my fountain-pen that my folks bought me. Gosh, I so hated to lose that but I was thankful that I didn't lose anything far greater than a pen. Since then, I've acquired a few "German" pens but they have no ink in them. I hope this letter will be mailed and censored in a hurry so that you'll receive it at the earliest possible moment.

[Friday] April 27th

Yesterday I was unable to write. I'm even not sure if whether I'll be able to finish this one before we move again and if I do I have no idea when I can mail it and when it will be censored but at least I'm making an effort to write.

Things are moving so fast that one never knows how long he'll be in one place. The night before last I did receive a package from my Dearest Darling. In the package were 2 cans of delicious fudge. Was that fudge made by Aunt Sally??

The sun is "peeking" its head out behind the clouds. It was raining practically the whole night but I believe it will clear up now.

[Saturday] April 28th

Gosh, but we had some nasty weather the last 24 hours. It's been raining hard since about 8 PM. I don't believe I'll ever "dry out" the way I feel now. Ha! Ha! Yesterday I hit the jackpot!! I received 13 letters!!

My Dearest, we wear the same shoes rain or shine!! No, they are not the same as the ones we wore in the states. They are known as "combat shoes".

[Sunday] April 29th

Today I experienced something new in the Army. The chaplain assigned permanently to our outfit is a Catholic Priest and naturally cannot conduct Protestant Services but he so much likes the Protestants to have church also. Previously when he couldn't get a Protestant chaplain one of the officers conducted our service but he was a war casualty so this noon he asked me if I'd conduct a Protestant Service. I could hardly refuse. By gosh, I'll bet there were about 75 or 100 men there. I said a few words, read a scripture lesson, sang some hymns. Lots of the fellows told me afterward they enjoyed the service.

[Monday] April 30th

Honey Dear, you are doing very well in saving money, in fact, I'm afraid you're "skimping" too much. Yes, my Dear is really becoming a wealthy woman lately. She is getting into "big" money!! Saving $20 in one week is very good. I'm proud of my wife, don't you forget that!!

[Wednesday] May 2nd

This is the first mail letter I've had a chance to write in over two weeks. I was told we can write the following story events. Of course, you'll probably know all about this by the time you receive this letter. We have now reached the foothills of the Alps. We've cleaned out the Po Valley[75], left the Apennines, and have reached the Alps. The 10th Division was the first outfit to cross the Po River[76] and that was an experience I'll never forget but all the details I'm afraid will have to wait until I get home. I can be thankful many, many times that I'm O.K., so you must not worry. You are probably anxiously waiting for mail from me right now and I hope that letter of the 25th travels real fast.

Yesterday and today thus far, I haven't received any mail. The day before yesterday I received seven letters, two from my Dear Wife and five from the folks up home. The letter you wrote on the 19th was marked as the 100th letter. I have such a fine and faithful wife. Always love me real, real much.

Yes, my Dearest, the baseball season is on. I haven't seen anything resembling a newspaper for the last five days so I can't tell you just how the teams are coming along. The last I saw the A's had a 4-2 record and were tied with Detroit for third place. The Phils were tied for last place with Pittsburg. Yes, my Sweetheart, I'll make a 50-cent bet with you. I'll take of course the St. Louis Cardinals to again win the National

---

[75] This a major geographical area of Northern Italy, a fertile valley, with the Po River running through it flowing east and emptying into the Adriatic Sea.

[76] The longest river in Italy and at its widest is 1,650 feet.

League Pennant. Now you pick the winner of the American League!!! Is that the kind of bet you had in mind??

R. Kauffman is getting his basic at Bainbridge, MD. That's a little closer to home than Great Lakes.

You and Sister don't seem to think Anita has made a particularly good selection!! Ha! Ha! Well, she probably thinks the same about your selection of a husband. How about it??? Yes, my Dear, I'm glad you sent me that picture of us "kissing"!! But you don't have to worry about me forgetting the techniques, I'm not that forgetful. Ha! Ha!

Yes, my Darling, that article you mentioned which appeared in "Life" [77] is just about how "patrolling" is done over here. Everything it must have said is true.

That indeed must have been mighty impressive at 4 PM (Sat. April 14th) [78] when everything and everybody came to a standstill while the church "chimes" were being played. Yes, it just seems impossible that our "great President" has passed on. Truman certainly has a big pair of shoes to fill.

That was my overseas jacket that I had on in that picture. Didn't you know that was the 10th Division insignia? I didn't have a "stripe" put on the jacket as yet. Time was so short and I didn't feel like wasting it by taking the time to have stripes sown on. That will all come later.

Gosh, but I'm sorry to hear that Grandpa sold that "lot" without first saying something to Father or us. Well, that's that. They probably thought we didn't want it since we didn't take it right away but I'm sorry for your Father's sake if he

---

[77] Life (magazine) was a weekly publication with a strong emphasis on photography. It was published from 1936 to 1972. The pictures it printed showed the stark reality of war to the American people.

[78] On this date President Roosevelt's funeral train arrived in Washington D.C. from Warm Springs, Georgia. Services were held in the East Room of the White House at 4 P.M.

had wanted to go into the "gas" business. That would have been fine to have his own Service Station.

[Thursday] May 3rd

I'm sure that by the time this letter reaches my Honey Bunch she will have heard the good news. Last night we heard that the war in Italy had been brought to an end. It was rather hard to believe, one doesn't want to get too over joyous and then be told later an error had been made, but it's seemingly official. Our Commanding General of the 10th Mt. Division, General Hays, has made an official announcement to all his troops. Gosh, but he spoke of his Division!! He said in part that he never saw or heard of an outfit that could come close to this Division. General Clark among other high officials really had high praise for the Division.

You know it still doesn't seem real that hostilities have ended in Italy. It still hasn't soaked in. The rumors are really "flying" now as to what we're going to do. We haven't heard anything definite as to what is happening on the Western and Eastern Fronts except that we're cutting Germany, Austria, and Czechoslovakia into many pieces, aren't we? I haven't seen a "Stars and Stripes" for a week now so we aren't sure of anything. We do know, of course, that Hitler and Mussolini are dead and we're not a bit sorry for that. Ha! Ha! Ha! You'd soon better be getting all those good dinners ready. Ha! Ha! Of course, I guess you'll have plenty of time to prepare all those meals!

You should have seen how the Partisans in this town were carrying on last night. They had a parade and were yelling and shouting like mad. They were hugging all the American soldiers they could. I presume there were some celebrations in the States also, weren't they??? Of course, I presume, hostilities have not ended in Germany as yet but I believe victory there is not far distant. We must crush Japan yet and then again, we'll have a world at Peace. Let's pray that the day is not far distant so that men and women the world over may return to their homes and live their lives in Peace.

I'm quite sure they must have published the American League Baseball schedule in either the "Times" or the "Eagle"!! Every other year that I can remember they published both schedules. The day they had it must have been a day my Honey didn't get to look at the paper. How about it??? I predict the A's will finish second or third this year. I guess you think I'm "crazy" for thinking that but that's my hunch. I'm afraid the Phils won't do better than seventh place and I doubt very much if they'll even get out of the cellar.

Ruth Dear, I wouldn't be surprised if that check of $99.57 you received did come from Howard's person. They probably got his money and made an effort to send that home first. If it was in his wallet, they probably would send that home with the rest of his personal belongings.

Yes, my Darling, we helped take those mountain peaks you mentioned and I know what the papers meant when they said we had "stiff" opposition. I thought "Belvedere" was rough but that was just a drop in the bucket compared to what we experienced lately. But it's over and I'm O.K. so why think of that. I can just be mighty thankful to Him for carrying me safely through.

Dear, you mustn't think that because everyone you show that picture of me to says it's such a good picture that it really is that good. They just say that to make you feel good, deep down they're saying it's a terrible picture. Ha! Ha!

Yes, the day we see each other again will be the biggest day of our lives, won't it?? But you mustn't let the war get on your nerves. Have faith and courage and I'm sure you'll feel lots better. Things look pretty good at the moment and I'm sure the final victory is not far away.

We've been getting pay quite regularly. I've received my pay up until the end of March. I haven't received April pay yet but we've been on the go so much that they just can't "hold up" the war just to pay the soldiers. Heavens, a fellow can't find an opportunity to spend it anyway.

[Friday] May 4th

They gave out some "Stars & Stripes" this morning and I see that the war news looks quite good on the European Side of the Universe. By gosh, all the large and industrious cities of the "Reich" have fallen into the hands of the Allies and I just believe it amounts to "mopping up" operations anymore. While the German resistance is disorganized in practically all sections, it is still quite bitter and fierce. We haven't moved for the last three days!!!

The death of President Roosevelt was indeed a great shock to me as it was to all our soldiers and folks the whole world over. There seems to be something missing. The world doesn't seem the same and to think some folks wanted to put him out of office last November. I too believe that Truman will do a better job than we first thought. I never liked him too much myself, but he might do better than expected. If peace comes and we will organize a strong international peace organization and he will follow through with Roosevelt's Domestic policies of 60,000,000 jobs after the war, which Henry Wallace can aid him in doing, I will feel very good.

You know Honey, you really must be quite "chilly" after all those "chills" you're having when you think of me coming home. Ha! Ha! You know, you mustn't think of that too much or you'll catch a cold from all those "chills". You know your hubby still is a great tease!!

Dearest, I never thought of bawling you out for not saving more money. You are doing very well. Naturally, I don't want my wife to spend money foolishly but I know she doesn't do that, so I'm not worrying.

Yes, Sister wrote in one of her letters that in the last letter Norman wrote home he mentioned me and was going to look me up. Why war must take all our best men I cannot see. You know when "Death" strikes a fellow you've been working close to and learned to know quite well it really hurts and I've experienced that many times lately.

Haven't you received those gifts I sent home from Florence yet? It's been almost five weeks. I'm sure you'll be very disappointed when you receive them because they won't be as nice as you thought they'd be.

Yes, my Darling, you can gladly join the Reformed Church. Do you think your parents would mind? It doesn't matter at all to me, you just do as you wish.

[Saturday] May 5th

Thanks, my dearest for enclosing the sports news. It's certainly interesting to notice the lineups of the major league teams and how they differ from last year. I don't believe anyone enjoys baseball like I do. I guess you think your honey is a "fanatic" in baseball, don't you??

I'm writing this letter by the light of a candle. We've moved again but for the first time in many weeks it was "back" instead of "forward". I'm sleeping in some kind of barn. It's not as nice as other places we were at but it suits me alright.

Sunday a week is Mother's Day. Gosh, honey, I'm afraid you'll have to do the shopping for both our Mothers alone.

We have the very best Mothers in all the world and we can't thank God enough for giving them to us.

[Sunday] May 6th

Last night, rather late, I received six letters and two boxes. One box contained four cans of the most delicious cookies with icing on them. Did Mother bake them? If so, you must thank her many, many times over for them. Everyone who had one commented on how good they were. The other box was from Grandmother and contained nothing but good pretzels. Gee whiz, did the fellows "dive" for them. After eating "C & K" rations for such a long spell you have no idea what such things as cookies and pretzels taste like! Ha! Ha!

What we are going to do remains a mystery but there are strong rumors that for a short time at least we'll have some kind of "training" program right here where we now are. What we're going to train for is beyond me. Ha! Ha! But what a relief not to have to hear those mortars and artillery shells "popping" all over the place. It seems that one has nothing to worry about anymore. Ha! Ha! There is a rumor circulating that the Germans in the European Theater are going to surrender unconditionally. Wow, what a rumor if true!!!! That really would be good news, wouldn't it???

Say, why didn't you go to see that movie "A Tree Grows in Brooklyn"?[79] I never heard of the movie or the book for that matter until you mentioned it but it sounds very interesting. Gosh, I hope my Dearest saw that picture that she

---

[79] This movie was about a poor but aspiring family of Irish decent in which James Dunn won the Academy Award for best supporting Actor. In 2010 the movie was selected to be preserved in the US National Film Registry.

said she'd like to see starring Spencer Tracy and Katherine Hepburn.

Dearest, how is that right eye of yours??? You told me that it was "pasted" shit in the morning and it was inflamed and there might have been a yellow spot on the eyeball. Honestly, my Darling, I'm so worried about your eyes. I'm only hoping and praying that it isn't an ulcer. If only I'd be home so that I could be sure you'd attend to it right away.

I guess I must call my wife an old "gossip"!! Why?? She stands in town talking for half an hour with other women discussing all the town news. How about it?? Ha! Ha! Just kidding, my Sweet!! You are really getting to be quite well known in the community of Leesport, aren't you?

Honey Darling, I guess I must agree with you that Mother cheats. I hate to have to admit it but if that is true what you say about her subtracting 35 instead of adding it and giving you the game why she must cheat. Ha! Ha! I must "tease" her about that. You must be the champion if you won two successive three-handed games. I always said my Honey was good in everything she did!!!

So, Linda is becoming a sweet young lady!! Well, I'm so glad to hear that. For a time she was quite annoying but when one thinks about it, you can easily picture her as becoming a very sweet and dignified person. With Michael what he is, Uncle Eddie has two very lovely children!! Is Michael still as cute and pleasant as he always was?

Here are the answers to your Questions of 3/28/45!! Answer to question I- 1) is supposedly the correct answer but when things get rough 2) is what really happens. Question II- 1) is the correct answer. Question III- That is a hard question to answer. We medics are not supposed to carry one. I don't. Question IV- I did mine by "foot". Did I answer all your questions satisfactorily???

Dearest, now that things are over in Italy and I'm sure you won't worry about me to the extent you had been I have some news to tell you that is indeed unpleasant for me to write as it is for you to read. I didn't know whether I should tell you or not but now that hostilities have ceased, I guess I should inform you. My good friend Ed has been a war casualty. It happened in the early part of this "push". I could hardly believe it but such are the fortunes of war. It hit pretty close to "home" when they got "Ed". Please don't worry about me. I'm very well and everything is under control now in Italy.

[Monday] May 7th

The Germans are surrendering on all fronts now.[80] I see yesterday all of their southern armies have surrendered to General Eisenhower.[81] I guess they finally realize that they can't fight anymore, that they are utterly defeated and disorganized. I guess you people are celebrating this good news,[82] aren't you?? Ha! Ha!

Yesterday afternoon we had church services at 2 PM along the Lake. We are situated along Lake Garda and it is very beautiful. It's considered the most beautiful spot in all of Italy, yes probably all of Europe. The town where Mussolini had his summer villa and where he spent his last days is right across the lake from where we are. The chaplain heard about

---

[80] Formal negotiations for Germany's surrender began at Reims, France with full surrender to the Allies on May 7th. Ceasefire took effect one minute after midnight May 8th. Truman stated "this solemn but glorious hour. I wish that Franklin D. Roosevelt had lived to see this day".

[81] Prior to becoming President in 1953, Dwight Eisenhower served during World War II as the Supreme Commander of the Allied Expeditionary Forces in Europe.

[82] Designated as V-E Day, Americans celebrated with waving flags and displaying the sign for victory. The Stars and Stripes newspaper printed "Prayers, tears, laughter- the world celebrates".

me conducting services the previous week and would like me to activate the Christian Service Men's League and now I'm supposed to organize and conduct its meetings. You know a good job to have in this man's army, the chaplain's assistant. What a position!! Ha! Ha!

Say, aren't you in jail yet for forging my name on that license application??? You know I filed an application to give you "Power of Attorney" but the form was not filled out correctly so now I don't know how things are.

That dog of yours, Flush, really must be a lively animal. She is tearing Mother's stockings and everything! Ha! Ha! Ha! Your Mother wrote in her letter that she is going to make out a bill for all the things that Flush is tearing and give it to you. Ha! Ha! You say the dog is changing color, is becoming a deeper red. It seems poor Judy is being neglected lately. I bet she's jealous when Flush gets so much attention. Now you must favor her sometimes to keep peace in the family. Ha! Ha! Ha!

Dearest, I see you are having a difficult time deciding about changing jobs. I can see where there seem to be lots of advantages for you by working for Mamie and yet a person hates to change jobs after working at a place as long as you have. Then too, you're sure of your job where you now are whereas can you be sure of steady employment at Temple. Whatever you decide on feel content and satisfied that you have done the right thing.

Yes, I can well remember April 1st, 1944. That was a "difficult" day to live through. So much has happened since then. Now I'm over here in Italy too. By golly, they didn't keep me in the states very long, did they??? Well, they needed good men over here to win the war and that's exactly what we did, didn't we??? Now, I'm not "bragging"!!! Am I??? Ha! Ha!

Dearest, you ask me about the towns in Italy!!! Florence is about the only city of any importance that I've been in, no our outfit did not go through Bologna. There are no huge Department Stores here like there are in the U.S.A. There are just small shops. Every shop sells one particular "line" of goods. The buildings as a rule are quite similar. I believe even the best homes do not come up to our average house.

I'll bet my Honey Bunch felt like a pig on Easter Sunday when she ate two meals. So, you had ham down-home. That's the typical Easter dish. Naturally, you should have eaten with your parents. It wouldn't at all have been the right thing to have them sit down to an Easter meal alone. Boy, that would have suited me just fine, having two meals in one day. That gives me an idea. When I come home, I think we'll have to eat dinner on Sunday at both our homes. That will help me catch up with all I'm missing. Ha! Ha! Yes, you should scold Mother for not going to communion on Easter. You say she was the only Kunkleman not present. I'm glad that your Grandfather was there.

[Tuesday] May 8th

We might be on the "move" again at any moment. You folks, I guess, were starting to celebrate the "Victory" last Saturday when the rumor was reported as fake. They should not report such things unless they are absolutely sure. It's too big a letdown.

So, my Sweetheart worked on the car. My but I bet you keep it "shined up". You'll put your husband to shame because it looked pretty dirty for me, didn't it?

[Wednesday] May 9th

We move again today. We are about 12 miles southwest of where we had been. We're in a small town in the foothills of the Alps. Starting tomorrow we'll inaugurate some kind of training schedule.

[Thursday] May 10th

My Dearest Snookums,

How do you like that for a salutation!!! I can see you're terribly worried. You haven't received any mail from me for a week and I'm afraid my letter won't reach you much before the 5th of May (the one of the 25th). I can feel assured, however, that by this time you are feeling quite good. First, because you're hearing from me and second because the European war is "finito". Isn't it a grand and glorious feeling that after all these years of war and killing there is at least peace in Europe?? Now to have Japan capitulate and then we really could celebrate!

Last night after I had finished your letter and received two letters, I still got a box of food. Before we went to bed a group of us fellows really "tore" into that box. This morning all that is left is the can of fruit cocktail and the cocoa. That fruit salad I'm going to save for a rainy day.

The building we are staying in was formally a schoolhouse. It's a huge building, two stories. We're sleeping on the floor of course, but even that is much better than a foxhole. The rumor has it that we will be issued cots. Gosh, I think I'll be living in style then. Ha! Ha!

Do you really think that we'll be able to retire by the time I get home? I guess you don't expect me home so early then because I don't think we can retire on what we have at the particular moment. All kidding aside my Honey Bunch is doing an excellent job saving our money.

Have you received my letter concerning that baseball bet??? Your suggestion about those bets suits me just fine. The last standing, I saw the Cards were tied with the Cubs for third place. Gosh, it makes me feel "sick" to see some ball games. Honey Bunch, when I first get back, I'll drag you to the ballpark 3 or 4 times a week. Do you mind??? Ha! Ha!

My sister tells me you're a swell gal. Yes, they all know how lucky I was to have received such a Dear and Wonderful Wife. She says that you are sorry, however, that you had to get such a "terrible" sister-in-law. Did you actually say that?? Ha! Ha!

[Friday] May 11th

Honey Bunch, in your letter of April 7th you tell me you should be praised for eating breakfast. Dear, I should bawl you out for not always eating breakfast. From this very day on you eat breakfast and that's an order.

[Saturday] May 12th

(Letter enclosed entitled-Headquarters 15th Army Group-3 May 1945)

PRESIDENTIAL MESSAGE

I take great pleasure in conveying to each American officer and enlisted man in the 15th Army Group the following message received by me from the President of the United States:

"ON THE OCCASION OF THE FINAL BRILLANT VICTORY OF THE ALLIED ARMIES IN ITALY IN IMPOSING UNCONDITIONAL SURRENDER UPON THE ENEMY, I WISH TO CONVEY TO THE AMERICAN FORCES UNDER YOUR COMMAND AND TO YOU PERSONALLY THE APPRECIATION AND GRATITUDE OF THE PRESIDENT AND OF THE PEOPLE OF THE UNITED STATES. NO PRAISE IS ADEQUATE FOR THE HEROIC ACHIEVEMENTS AND MAGNIFICENT COURAGE OF EVERY INDIVIDUAL UNDER YOUR

COMMAND DURING THIS LONG AND TRYING
CAMPAIGN"
"AMERICA IS PROUD OF THE ESSENTIAL
CONTRIBUTION MADE BY YOUR AMEICAN ARMIES
TO THE FINAL ALLIED VICTORY IN ITALY. OUR
THANKS FOR YOUR GALLANT LEADERSHIP AND
THE DEATHLESS VALOR OF YOUR MEN".
HARRY S. TRUMAN
MARK W. CLARK
General, USA Commanding

(Enclosed is also a black and white postcard of Riva del
Garda[83]-
Panorama. Written on the back:
This is the town we were situated in when the Germans
surrendered in Italy. It didn't look quite like this when we
were there.)

[Saturday] May 12th
How do you like my red ink? My pen was dry and I saw a
bottle of this red ink and mine was in my pack so I decided to
try it. We are having a training schedule that we are following
so I don't have any time to write during the day. We do not
have such a good lighting system so my time for letter-
writing is cut rather short. I'm made to understand that
censorship rules have been relaxed somewhat so I'll probably

---

[83] This is a town on the northwest corner of Lake Garda in Northern Italy.
There is a medieval belfry/clock tower "Torre Apponale" built before
1273. The tower is open to the public; around 160 steps to the top with
great views.

write more freely. We're in a town called Caprino.[84] Rumor has it that we'll only be here about 4 or 5 more days.

This morning we had about 1 1/2 hours of calisthenics and close order drill and then we took a "hike" of about 2 hours. This afternoon we're supposed to have an hour of orientation and two hours of Mass Athletics. Boy, that sun is hot again today.

You naturally know that I was at Camp Patrick Henry[85] after leaving Camp Swift. We arrived there on Christmas Eve at about 8:30. It was a nasty dreary night too. I'll never forget it. We boarded the U.S.S West Point[86] at New Port News on Wednesday, Jan 3rd at about 6 PM. We stayed in the harbor until about 11 AM Thursday when we pulled out with bands playing and flags waving. Ha! Ha! The West Point was a huge ship. We pulled into Naples, Italy on Saturday the 13th around 7 PM. We remained on the ship until 11 AM Sunday where we transferred to LCI boats (Landing Craft Infantry), eight of them in all. We headed North along the Italian Coast. We hit Leghorn (Livorno)[87] at about 2 PM Monday. I'll continue at a later date.

Yes, Honey, you don't have to send me any "Baked Beans" for I'm really full of beans. So many cans of "C" rations contained beans in one sort or another. Florence is a nice city all right but it is nothing to compare to our cities. Probably in the prewar days, it was really beautiful.

---

[84] This is a municipality in the Province of Verona, about 75 miles from Venice.

[85] Located in Warwick County, Virginia it served as a staging ground for troops going overseas. At its peak in could house around 35,000 people.

[86] In 1941 this ship was painted camouflage gray and converted to a troop transport with a capacity of over 7,000 soldiers.

[87] This Italian city know in English as "Leghorn" is a port city on the coast of Tuscany. It suffered extensive damage during the war with many historic sites destroyed.

173 people weren't too many for a spring communion. Do you think? We often ran over 200, but we must remember that many of the young men have entered the service. You're darn right we are going to go bicycle riding when I get home. We both enjoy that very much. Yes, your parents certainly are "spry" for their age. You really must admire them for that. They have more pep than we young folks have.

No, my Dear, I haven't seen any Japanese-American troops. They are on the west coast of Italy. Yes, they fought very, very well. Their Regiment has done remarkably well throughout the whole war.

(Enclosed also is a letter entitled: 27 April 1945)

Headquarters Fifty Army

To: See Distribution

1. The following message has been received from the Commanding General, 15th Army Group:

"Please convey to all ranks of the Fifth Army my heartiest congratulations on your successful drive which has taken you beyond the Po River. Your troops began their offensive faced with the difficult task of driving the enemy from strongly held mountain defenses. They rapidly overcame these obstacles and forged ahead to and beyond Bologna. With Bologna in our hands, the Po was our next objective. Without delay, our troops pushed on to reach and cross it. All elements of your command have performed magnificently in this action. Your units spearheaded by the gallant 10th Mountain Division have dealt the enemy a staggering blow. The 10th Mountain Division, which entered the line only last January, has performed with outstanding skill and strength. I am confident that you will press forward relentlessly until you have destroyed the enemy.

2. To the above commendation of the Army Group Commander, I desire to add my congratulations and deep appreciation of the heroic manner in which all members of the Fifth Army and XXII Tactical Air Force surged out into the Po Valley after the long winter in the mountains. The coordination and energy you put into the attack have carried across the Po Valley to the foot of the Alps. You passed two major river obstacles in stride. In twelve days, you have broken the German Army in two and scattered the forces that had spent the entire winter constructing defenses and preparing to meet your attack.

3. The enemy now seeks to delay our advance while they reassemble their broken and scattered forces in the mountains to the North. You have them against the ropes, and it now remains for you to keep up the pressure, the relentless pursuit and enveloping tactics to prevent their escape, and to write off as completely destroyed the German Armies in Italy.

4. Now is the time for speed. Let no obstacle hold you up, since hours lost now may prolong the war for months. The enemy must be completely destroyed here. Keep relentlessly and everlastingly after them. Cut every route of escape, and complete victory will be yours.

L.K. Truscott, Jr.

Lieutenant General, U.S.

Army Commanding

[At the bottom of this letter]

Distribution:

Headquarters, 10th Mountain Division, APO 345, U.S. Army, 3 May 1945

To: Officers and Men, 10th Mountain Division, APO 345, U.S. Army

You may all take pride in the above official recognition of the part we played in the final defeat and destruction of the cruel and vicious Nazi forces in Italy.

George P. Hayes

Major General, US Army Commanding

[Sunday] May 13th

This morning at 8:30 we were told how many "points"[88] we had with a reference to getting a Discharge. "By Jiminy", I need quite a few more to get out of this Army. It probably doesn't mean anything anyway. As I said before, you never know where you are at in the Army. Ha! Ha! None of my buddies came close to having enough points either. The average number of points is low. At 10:00 we had church services and the chaplain had a very fine Mother's Day Service. He asked before he started his sermon how many of us were able to spend last Mother's Day with their Mother's and very few raised their hands.

Let me continue where I left off in yesterday's letter concerning my adventures since I left the States. We remained on the L.C.I.s until about 2 PM, then we were loaded on trucks and driven to a "staging area" on the outskirts of Pisa. There we slept in pup tents. One night I managed to slip into Pisa and saw the "leaning tower". That's the only thing I wanted to see. You know that is one of the seven wonders of the world and I'm telling you there isn't anything phony about that. It leans 12 feet from the top to the bottom. That was something to see. We remained at this staging area until Friday the 19th of January. We left there by trucks and were driven to a small town in the Apennines

---

[88] This was officially the "Advanced Service Rating Score" which boiled down to "those who fought longest and hardest should be returned home for discharge first". Enlisted men needed a score of 85 to be considered.

called Prunetta.[89] It was quite a drive and we stopped along the way and all the trucks were ordered to put on their chains. Soon after that, we started climbing and gosh, did we run into snow. The truck I was in got into a bank and we had quite a time until we got out. Prunetta was having a lot of snow during that part of January. Before I go any further let me explain just what outfit I'm in. I'm, of course, part of the 15th Army Group, of which the 5th Army is a part. Next, of course, I'm in the 10th Mt. Division which consists of three Regiments, the 85th, 86th, and 87th, Infantry Regiments. I'm in the 85th Regiment. Now the "Regiment" is divided into three Battalions; 1st, 2nd, and 3rd. I'm, of course, in the 3rd Battalion and as a Medic was attached to Co. I of the Battalion (also Co. L for a while). Again, I'll stop telling you my travels and experiences and continue them in a later letter. I've just been told we are moving in a day or two. Where I don't know!!

My Dearest, in our Med Detachment we have two officers, an M.C. (Doctor) and a M.A.C. The M.C. takes care of all the Medical work attached to the unit while the M.A.C. is supposed to "run" and administer the Detachment.

Does my Dearest Honey Bunch think I'll spend all of the holidays in 1946 at home? Yes, let's hope that is true. We've defeated one of our enemies and now the Jap is the only one we must overrun. The war over here certainly did take a favorable turn in the last month, didn't it?? Yes, I too hope we'll spend our future holidays, together. I'm so anxious to know what we're in for. I understand that where we're going, we'll be living in our pup tents.

Speaking of that large building where we stayed when I was in Florence, I'll tell you what it was. It was a huge

---

[89] A province of Pistoia located 169 miles North West of Rome with an elevation of over 3,000 ft.

railroad depot and a hotel attached. Yes, it really was some huge building. I didn't feel as though I wanted any of these jewelers over her to work on my watch any more than necessary. In the first place they might not do a good job on it and then too, they know how to "charge" so I figure while she still is running as well as she does, I won't let anybody touch it. I'll have it cleaned thoroughly when I get home.

When you come to think of it the mail service is wonderful. I believe we get all our mail both you people and myself. It's amazing, isn't it??

Yes, my Sweet, we have given Blood Plasma right on the front lines at times. When the man is losing too much blood, I administer it right away. As a rule, we Medics are responsible for a certain group of men but when things get "rough" in combat you help one another out.

As I'm sitting writing this letter here in a building, I'm starting to sweat so you can imagine how hot it is over here in Italy. Ha! Ha! your "hubby" still does quite a bit of "sweating" as you can still see. I can well remember how I perspired at Barkeley. I was ringing wet day and night.

[Monday] May 14th

Oh, I'm always so glad when I find time to write to my good wife. As you can see, I wasn't able to get to writing until quite late today. That's right, you guessed it again. We moved to a "bivouac" area about 40 miles south. I've heard we'll be here from four to six weeks.

Haven't you received those gifts I sent from Florence yet???

[Tuesday] May 15th

Gosh, but I'm at a loss to know how I'm going to write all my letters. You know it takes me quite a while to write these "long" letters and I can't find any more time during the day because they keep you busy from morning until supper. Since we're living in pup tents it's quite difficult to write after dark although I managed to "hook" a small piece of a candle to write with after dark. Ha! Ha! Gosh, but it's hot again today. I'm "ringing wet".

Boy, it's amazing how quickly Army life has changed since the war has ended over here and especially since we've moved into this last area. It's getting to be the same as when you were back in the States. You must always be in a proper uniform. You must salute all officers. You must be in your "bunk" by a certain time. We're going to have an equipment and clothing inspection tomorrow, I think, and also a Divisional parade.

Let's continue again from where I left off in Sunday's letter. We were in Prunetta for one week. While there we took various hikes in the mountains and gosh that was something with all that snow on the ground. Well on the 26th of January we moved. It was about 11 PM that Friday night when trucks came along for us. Of course, things were rather quiet then in the 5th Army section. We hit our destination at about 3 AM Saturday. That same morning about 11:00 a few of us were selected to go up farther. We went to a town called Cutigliano. We reached there

Saturday afternoon. We stayed in this town for quite some time. On Sunday night Co. I sent out a patrol to capture some high ground near the town which was held by the Germans. They ran into some "action" and one man was killed. It was a coincidence his name was "Schneider" and when the Med. Dept. first heard that a Schneider was killed, they thought it was I since they knew I was up there. That mountain was rough. It was icy and you had to be careful or you'd hit the "tripwires". The boy was shot and there wasn't much that could be done except stopping the flow of blood. He died the next morning. That was our first casualty. That's what I experienced on January 28th, 1945. Again, I'll stop at this point and continue in a later letter. Ok???

I have before me my Darling a V-Mail letter of yours which was written on April 13th, the day after President Roosevelt died. As I mentioned before, we found it out about 7 AM the morning of the 13th and you'll never know how funny a feeling I had. I knew that the next morning we were going to start on our "big" push and gee, I really had an "empty" feeling. It seemed as though something was taken from our lives. Everyone had words of praise and good feelings for him. I guess my Father took it rather hard. He admired him so very much. Well, he'll go down in history as one of the greatest Presidents we've ever had. He did more for the average man than any President we've ever had! When things were on the "rocks" in 1933 when he entered office, he restored faith and a good feeling in the populace for the government and democracy. He was great in peace and war, a trait a very few Presidents ever had.

My Dearest, I still insist on paying you all those bills of ours you are now paying no matter what you say. You know that even though I'm not at home at present to take care of things is no reason why I should still not be responsible for them, so remember that. I want you to keep a note of all the money you've spent on us. Now please, please do that. You'll make your "hubby" very, very happy. Will you please listen to me???

So, Mother tells Granma to go ahead and bid because she has all the 13s. Ha! Ha! And you think that is cheating??? Yes, I must agree with you on that!! I'm beginning to believe that everyone cheats except Grandma. I honestly don't believe Grandma cheats but Mother is constantly telling me that you and Sister cheat. Ha! Ha! I can see quite a few changes that must be made when I return home.

Dearest, you mention sending more "requests"!!! With conditions so unsettled now and not knowing where we're going or what we're going to do, I won't request anything. As soon as we know what we're going to do and when we're settled, I'll request a lot of things again.

[Wednesday] May 16th

I didn't receive any mail yesterday but this afternoon I hit the jackpot. I got seven letters in all!!! Among your letters was the one you wrote on May 4th and gosh it made me feel just as happy to know you heard from me as it did you. Thanks a lot for including the baseball standings. You know, I guess, how much that interests me.

[Thursday] May 17th

We saw a movie today entitled "Two Down and One to Go".[90] It must be shown to every officer and enlisted man in the Army. You can imagine what it was about by the title. I mentioned a few days ago that we were told that censorship had been relaxed somewhat and as a result, I was beginning to relate my experiences while in Italy. Well, yesterday we were told that all unit censorship would again go into effect. Things are very uncertain. You don't know from one hour to the next what you'll be doing or where you'll be.

Say my Sweetness, what do you mean by saying that if I don't soon request food you are going to give me the "works" when I get home??? Now you must clarify that statement

---

[90] This was a motivational film celebrating the enemy defeat in Africa and Europe but still having to defeat Japan. It was produced in Technicolor and ended with the "Star Spangled Banner".

more than you have. I'm just too "dumb" to know what that means. Ha! Ha!

Honey, I really must laugh and laugh some more when I read and recall in my mind what happened to you on Sunday, May 6th when the car got hot and then to "top" if off you locked the keys in the car. Remember how I did that once and Howard and I worked for about an hour until finally we got a wire in through the ventilator and opened it that way. Thanks, my sweet, for sending me the Times Baseball News of Monday the 6th. Boy, Kurowski[91] really went to town on Sunday didn't he or doesn't my Sweet follow sports anymore? She better had or I'll disown her. Ha! Ha! Just kidding.

Gosh but I'm sorry to hear that your tomato plants were frozen. How are the cabbage plants coming along?? It's too bad that it had to get that cold after being so nice and warm.

Well, I guess now my Wife wants me to buy another car after the war. Ha! Ha! So, you drove another car that had a "hydramatic"[92] drive. I've seen them already but I'm not sure I ever drove one. From what I've heard before and what you say it really must be easy to drive.

[Saturday] May 19th

It's very unusual for me to be writing in the afternoon but I'm on K.P. today and we finished our pots and pans around 1:00 and the cook told me I could take off until 4:00. I didn't know I would be on K.P. until 6:45 today. I was unable to write yesterday. We're about 7 Km. from a rather large town and some men naturally go in. Now, this might seem peculiar

---

[91] "Whitey Kurowski, a native from Reading, Pa. played 3rd base for St. Louis.

[92] Hydramatic drive was a semi-automatic transmission that required the driver to clutch shift in and out of gear but not between the two forward gears. In 1939 this option costing $57 was first offered on Oldsmobiles.

to you but some soldiers are attracted to Italian girls and you know what takes place!! Ha! Ha! Well, we "medics" established a "prophylactic" station in town for these men as a guard against V.D. We operate it from 6 to 11 PM and it came to my turn. What a job!!! Ha! Ha! As a result, my time was occupied the whole day.

My Darling, I'm quite sure we're going to leave this area tomorrow and I believe we're going quite a distance so I'm doubtful whether I'll be able to write. You folks have really gone "hysterical" since you heard what Fulton Lewis said. Now you must not build too high hopes of me coming home soon. I'm not saying that I won't get a furlough but I also know nothing of the fact that I will. What he referred to I believe is "medics" that are not attached to any combat unit. I think he meant "hospital" medics. You see we'll travel with the 10th Mt. Division. If the Division goes home, we'll go home.

Yes, the Boston Red Sox had a hard time getting started, didn't they?? I don't believe they'll finish higher than 6th place. I'm rather disappointed with "athletics". They are 6th now and I still believe they'll end up in the first division. That Russ Christopher, their ace pitcher, is pitching a good ball. Our Phillies are in their usual position, aren't they?? They certainly would surprise everyone if they'd happen to have a good team one year. Ha! Ha! Gosh, they don't have any one of any account!!! My Honey is going to be tired of sports after I've dragged her to every event for a radius of 100 miles. Well, there isn't any finer or cleaner entertainment than sports. We'll all eat plenty of Hot Dogs and soda pop. Ha! Ha! Ha!

Dearest, I'm so glad you enjoyed that movie "A Song to Remember".[93] I see Sister won the argument you had said in a previous letter that you would have rather seen "Van Johnson" at the Lowes. Wouldn't Sister go along there or did she convince you that the Embassy was the better picture? Mother sent me $10.00 as a V.E. Day present and the program of the V.E. Day Service from May 8th. That was the first $10.00 bill I've seen in over four months.

[Monday] May 21st

Dearest, don't look for a letter from the 20th; I said we were moving a long distance and that's exactly what we did. We moved by trucks and a good 175 or more miles. I can't tell you where we are but if you follow the controversies which are at "high pitch" in and around Northern Italy you have guessed where I am. Who knows, I might see other countries besides Italy before I leave Europe. We're living in pup tents again and my partner's the same fellow as before. He's the fellow who married a girl from Allentown and is a darn nice fellow. We traveled last night for about 4 hours, but I had a seat all the way and the scenery was beautiful.

Sweetheart, there seemed to be something worrying you in the last letter. You say your nerves were so jumpy and that you went for a walk during your lunch hour and they were a lot calmer after you got back. What's the matter, Dear? Is there something on your mind??? Now please my Sweet, tell me if anything worrying you. Now please do that for your "hubby's" sake!! Please when you fail to get a letter don't let it worry you or make you feel ill because I was just too busy to write those days. My Dear says she felt weak and sick in

---

[93] This is a 1945 Columbia Technicolor biographical film about the pianist and composer Frederic Chopin staring Paul Muni, Cornel Wilde, Merle Oberon and Nina Foch.

her stomach when she didn't get a letter. Now always remember that your "hubby" is O.K. and you never have anything to worry about. Now be a good girl and listen to your hubby!!!!

My wife had another nice dream the other night about walking through Leesport with her hubby. I too dream such things and then wake up and find myself about 4 to 5 thousand miles from home "burns" me up. Oh well, I say to myself then "my turn will come" and the longer I have to wait the more I'll appreciate that day.

Those poor Phillies are having a difficult time winning some games, aren't they??

[Tuesday] May 22nd

At 12:30 PM we were taken down the road a few miles to a shower unit where we had good hot showers. Gosh, did that feel good, I'm really very clean. We got all clean clothing. Just as I was ready to leave the tent it started to rain and of course we rode in an open truck so you can imagine how soaking wet we got. Well, such is life! Ha! Ha!

This is the third day that I haven't received any letters. I did get another package and the food tasted so very good. I and my buddies enjoyed the food while the thunderstorm was progressing. Everything is gone except for the sausages and I'm saving them for a real "rainy" day. Boy, are they going to taste good!!! This morning Med. Detachment and Headquarters Co. challenged each other in a game of softball and they chose me as the umpire. Well, I hate to say this but Medics lost pretty badly.

Your Father had quite a long day on Saturday, April 28th, I didn't remember him working until 11 PM for a long time, especially on a Saturday. Were they having inventory or some special order they had to get out?? Gee, I'm pretty inquisitive, aren't I??? Be sure and don't ask Father, or he'll think I'm rude. It isn't any of my business.

We are still having hot weather but tonight there is a cool breeze blowing and I hope I'll be able to sleep well. Before I go to bed, I must take a "hump" out of my bed. The ground is a little "lumpy" where I sleep and it annoyed me a bit last night.

I know that my Wife gave an excellent prayer again on Mother's Day. Yes, it was declared a National Day of Prayer to celebrate VE Day. We both are very lucky to have two such wonderful Mothers, aren't we???

So, you didn't know that you married such a "tough" man, did you?? Well to be perfectly honest with you, I didn't know either that I was that tough. I'm not going to be so hard on my Darling when I get home. Ha! Ha!

I think every American soldier will realize what the 10th Mt. Division did. I was told that this Division has received the Presidential Citation although that seems almost too good to be true. I know that Major General Hays is trying to get it for the outfit. Every man in the outfit will get it if the order comes through.

(Enclosed in the May 22nd letter)

HEADQUARTERS- 10TH MOUNTAIN DIVISION- APO 345, US ARMY

18 May 1945 To the Officers and Enlisted Men of the 10th Mountain Division

CITATION-- On the 16th of May the Division Commander, 10th Mountain Division was awarded the Distinguished Service Medal by the Commanding General, Fifth Army. The citation for this decoration is reproduced below. The decoration although awarded to the Division Commander was earned by the combined efforts of each officer and enlisted man in the entire division. Official recognition of the part played by the 10th Mountain Division is the decisive defeat of the German Armies in Italy is a source of pride to all.

George P. Hayes, 07149, Major General, United States Army

For exceptionally meritorious service in a duty of great responsibility from 24 December 1944 to May 1945, in Italy. Under General Hay's unusually competent supervision, the 10th Mountain Division established record time in its movement from the port of embarkation into line operations. The system used in equipping and moving this division is an outstanding tribute to the exceptionally efficient planning of General Hays. Major General Hays brilliantly led his Division through winter operations and during the spring offensive which culminated in the final triumph by the 15th Army Group over the German armies in Italy. After skillfully directing his troops in their first attack on Mount Belvedere and adjacent ridges, he committed his division to the task of spearheading the Allied drive through the Apennine Mountains, across the Po River Valley, and into the foothills of the Alps leading to the Brenner Pass. During these operations, the 10th Mountain Division, guided and directed by the ceaseless efforts of Major General Hays, distinguished itself by being the first element to breach the heavily fortified and extensively mined German line in the Apennines, by being the first division to cut strategically important Highway 9, and being the first element to cross the Po River. The leadership, aggressiveness, and sound tactical judgment of Major General Hays, together with outward manifestations of pride and confidence in his officers and men, can be attributed to the success of his Division's operations. His capable and loyal service in a position of great responsibility is in keeping with the highest traditions of the Army of the United States.

Jefferson J. Irvin

Lt. Col. GSC Chief of Staff

[Wednesday] May 23rd

I'm not sure I can tell you exactly where we are but I'm anxious that you know about the place. As you know by the papers some controversies are arising between the Allied Armies and Marshall Tito and his forces. Well at the moment our Division is occupying the territory which is so much in dispute. We are going to stay here I'm told until this matter is settled. We are trying to settle it diplomatically so I'm sure nothing will develop from it all.

Well, my Honey Bunch, they just gave me a copy of some general orders that came through Division and I see I was awarded the "Bronze Star"[94] for "Heroic achievements against the enemy in action on April 15th, 1945 at Castel D'aino. Well, that gives me five more points toward my discharge. Ha! Ha! Now don't go thinking your hubby is a hero now. I'm sure anyone in my shoes would have done the same thing but I happened to be there, so naturally, I just did my duty as I saw it. They give those "stars" supposedly for the Meritorious and Heroic achievements in combat. They say the medal you get is quite nice. You also get some sort of ribbon that you wear. I was hoping they'd award the "star" to Ed posthumously, but I see they didn't. He certainly must have done good work. I still can't see what I did that deserved

---

[94] This decoration is awarded by Captains of a Company or Battery to soldiers under their command who have displayed heroic deeds during a military operation. This award was designed by Rudolf Freund of Baily, Banks and Biddle. It's a bronze- colored star with 9 smaller stars in the center, hanging off a red ribbon with a blue strip in the middle.

the citation but I'll take it now that they gave it to me. Ha! Ha!

Ruth, dearest, how is your Mother's Rheumatism??? Gosh, I'm sorry to hear that she has that aliment!! It's so painful and annoying. Mother has arthritis and that too is so painful!!

Now my Dear, didn't you promise me many, many times that you wouldn't bite your fingernails anymore and here you go and bite them anyway. Honey Bunch, you seem to have so much trouble with headaches lately. Do you think it's your eyes?? Now please you must go to a doctor if you continue to be plagued with those things. Understand??? Now that's an order from your husband!!! You must listen to your hubby!! Thanks a lot, my sweet, for sending me the sport's standings every day. I enjoy them so very, very much.

I have before me the letter you wrote on May 1st and oh my but my Sweetheart was worried. She was so "blue" and I only wish I could have done something for her but I know by this time she feels much better. It was perfectly alright for you to take the day off but you must not worry because when you worry, I too feel bad and it makes things much worse for all of us.

[Thursday] May 24th

What a day this has been. Just about 4 PM a terrific thunderstorm came up and we couldn't keep the water out of our tent. I managed to keep the blankets dry but most of the ground inside the tent got wet. We had it "ditched" but apparently not deep enough for the ditches filled up and overflowed into our tent. I "ditched" it a little better and then had to get the ground as dry as possible before I spread the blankets. It's thundering right now and I'm afraid we'll get more rain before the nights over.

Last night we had mail call and I received that wonderful picture. Oh, Darling, I'm so happy. I look at it every spare moment I possibly can. I carry it in my shirt pocket next to my heart. Gosh, you look so wonderful, I can't find words to express how good it made me feel.

[Friday] May 25th

The latest rumor has us leaving here by the 27th (Sunday). Yes, this outfit moves on a Sunday practically all the time. We've nicknamed it the "Sunday Division". Ha! Ha!

Oh my, but I'm so glad you sent me that picture. I'm looking at it all the time and everyone asks who that lovely woman is and I stick out my chest and tell them that's my wife.

I'm enclosing in this letter a map showing you the area which is in dispute with regards to Tito and other Allied armies. You notice on the map a city called Udine. We are located at this moment about 7 miles directly east of Udine. I indicated our position with a "dot". Of course, we won't even be here anymore when you receive this letter. Ha! Ha! We were told again that censorship rules have been relaxed so I'll continue my story of some weeks back. I believe I stopped when we were in Cutigiano after that patrol where one man was killed. Well, we stayed in that vicinity until the 5th. Various patrols were sent out by the three companies but I as a medic did not go out with them until the 3rd of Feb. That night a group of men selected from the whole Battalion which added up to the strength of a company was going on a raiding party which included the taking of a high peak called La Serra. I was one of the medics scheduled to go along. We left LD (Line of Departure) at 1 AM on the 4th of Feb. We were all dressed in those white parkas because the snow was quite deep. Well, we reached the top of La Serra by dawn and set up our positions and then the mortars started landing in and golly they kept you busy all day fixing up wounded men. They hit so close one time I surely thought it would get me but I was fortunate enough to be missed. What a day that was! Late in the afternoon, our Commanding Officer got word to withdraw his forces and so we did. I helped to evacuate some wounded too since the whole company retreated. About six men were either killed or missing in action and quite a few were wounded. That night about 8 or 9 o'clock I wrote you that V Mail in which I told you I was so tired and believe me I was really tired. On the following day, the 5th, we returned to our town of Prunetta and we remained there for nearly two weeks. We took a shower while we were there, that is we were taken from there to a shower unit in a place called Campo Tizzoro. While at Prunetta we slept on cots and did some sort of training program until we left on the evening of Feb. 18th (Sunday again). I'll stop here until a later letter.

I never thought of the fact that soon Sister will have completed a full school term as a teacher at a University. She has certainly made good as a teacher. We can feel proud of her, don't you think?? I almost forgot!!! On Wednesday I also received a letter from Carpenter Steel in which was enclosed a check for $1.84 as payment of dividend for that Group Health and Accident Insurance which you carry at the plant. The letter states I should cash the check as soon as possible, so I'll endorse the check and enclose it in this letter.

You mentioned in your letter of May 3rd that one of the waitress's brother came home from Italy and that he was in the 12th Air Force. Well, those fellows really deserve a lot of credit in our final victory. They pounded the "Krauts" with machinegun fire and "rocket" bombs continuously. They set fire to their vehicles and ammunition dumps. Yes, the Air Force has done a wonderful job in this war.

Ever since I lost my fountain pen, I've been using this German pen. It writes quite well but doesn't hold as much ink. Well, Honey, we've taken quite a few prisoners and since it was through them, I lost my pen I happened to appropriate one or so for myself. You're not mad at me, are you?? They were willing to give them to me so I really didn't "steal" them. Knowing the German language helps a fellow get along with the "Krauts". I must laugh when I read your letter of May 4th after you had received my letter of April 25th. You say you enjoyed your lunch again and you were sure you were going to sleep well that night. Gosh, but my Honey must certainly have been happy that day, wasn't she??

[Saturday] May 26th

This has been another rapidly moving day thus far. This morning when we got up the sky was cloudy again and we just got our pup tents straightened out when the rains came. Well, it rained hard practically the whole morning but we managed to keep the water out of the tent and that was a miracle. Our ditches really worked today. Afternoon meal I was relaxing in my tent when my partner and I were asked to set up and run a prophylactic station in town about two miles east of where we are. This being a Saturday afternoon and evening they're afraid such a station is necessary. At the moment I'm writing in this "station" (we have a room in an Italian hospital in this town). We are on duty until 11 PM. So far, I haven't had any business and I hope I don't get any. I've heard this is a very "clean" town but the Doctor doesn't want to take any chances.

Well, I guess I'll continue now where I left off. Well, we found out on the 11th that the following week we were going to take Mt. Belvedere. So, we had a practice run that previous week. By that I mean they took us to some terrain which was a lot like Mt. Belvedere and we went through the same tactical movements that we were going to go through when we attack Mt. Belvedere. We left on this practice run on Monday morning Feb. 12th. We took positions that afternoon at an assembly point some distance from the "practice" mountain that we were going to climb. Well, the officers agreed the men understood thoroughly how we were going to "attack" Mt. Belvedere so about noon Tuesday we took off back to Prunetta. All Monday, and that night it was raining and cold. Gosh, I thought that experience was rough but that turned out to be nothing at all compared to what came the following week on Belvedere. Well from that Tuesday until the following Sunday at 7 PM when we left Prunetta we had some training and plenty of orientation on the coming attack at Belvedere. I'll leave here and continue later. Okay???

Honey Bunch, I have before me this very moment the letter you wrote on Monday, May 7th and I just re-read it and you guessed it perfectly, I'm having a good laugh over it. First of all, I'm laughing at you locking the keys in the car and then my Snookums thought she had walked ten miles when she actually didn't walk more than 2 miles. Then too, I must pity my Dear because she ran into so much trouble with the car. But you really must have had some experience that Sunday night. You most certainly did the wise thing by not driving it back home once she was so "hot".

[Sunday] May 27th

Last night till I got back from the "pro" station and got to bed it was midnight. I didn't sleep so very well so this morning after breakfast I dozed off till about 10:30 AM. Was I a bad boy now? Gosh, but I was so sleepy. Yesterday noon we were issued ties again so now whenever you're in your ODs you must wear a tie. Gosh, it seems so hot around your neck after not wearing one for such a long time.

Please, please don't you or your Father worry about that "cracked cylinder" head on the Chevy. Those things just happen sometimes and how we don't know. Now don't run yourself short of money. Just get some from the bank in case you don't have enough. $22.00 isn't too much for a new cylinder head, I don't think!! No Darling, I know you take excellent care of the car and it wasn't your fault at all, and tell your Father that it shouldn't bother him either because it certainly was no fault of his. You people worry about such little things. Nothing is important except that we are well.

At 2 PM we had worship services and it certainly was a very fine service, we even had communion. You know it makes a fellow real close to "God" when he takes communion in the open field.

Honey Darling, are you under the impression that we soldiers must pay our way home from Europe if we get furloughed?? If we get furloughed it would be only when we hit the U.S., understand?? And don't worry I'm having enough money saved for that if and when that time comes. Darling, you must not get so "hilarious" when you hear such reports as Fulton Lewis Jr. reported, and likewise do not be discouraged if you hear we're going directly to the South Pacific. No one knows exactly what we'll do.

My Dearest, that was so very thoughtful of your Father and you to fetch Grandma and Sister on V-E Day. I certainly can well understand how you must have felt and also your Father at a service such as that. You have no idea how often I think of Howard. It seems as though it just can't be so. I've seen so many "fall" and never "rise" again and one can see how "devastating" war is. We can say and keep in our minds the fact that they all died so others might live and live in freedom. I've lost quite a few close friends and that hurts especially when they're killed less than a foot from where you are and that happened many a time. We must just believe that such was their destiny and that "God" is taking care of all of them. They are not suffering but instead are in very good hands.

[Monday] May 28th

Honey Darling, for the last couple of days, five medics from our Battalion can go on a 24hr. pass to Venice, Italy every day, and tomorrow I'm slated to go. You get up at 4:30 and get back around midnight. The Army takes you and brings you back. It's almost 100 miles from here so it'll be a long ride but Venice is the city of canals and gondolas so since I have the opportunity, I guess I'd better go. Does my Dearest mind too much??? I'm afraid I won't get a chance to write tomorrow, so don't get alarmed. Am I forgiven??? I understand that the army sponsors "tours" in the city itself. Venice you know is along the Adriatic coast of Italy. I'll tell you all about it in my Wednesday letter.

Let me continue my activities from Feb. 18th at 7 PM. We left Prunetta by truck and drove for about three hours. At about 10 PM we disembarked and started walking and what a terrible walk that was. I had a terribly heavy load on my back and the hike was upgrade the whole way and you'd sink in the mud almost up to your knees and that is no exaggeration. Well, we finally hit our destination for the night at about 3 AM Monday. Then we dug in for the night!!! That whole day Monday we were told to rest as much as possible because we'd be on the move that coming night. Well, they weren't kidding us either!!! At 10 PM we left this assembly area and took off for our Line of Departure. Co I was supposed to come up Mt. Belvedere on the right and Co. L, on the left, and Co. K was supposed to support Co. I because they thought they'd encounter the most difficulty. Well, we made our way up the mountain peak amid small arms fire and as we were approaching the real slopes the "Krauts" let us have everything but the "kitchen sink". What an ordeal those next few hours were. All you'd hear was "Medic", "Medic"! It was horrible!!! You'd see shells land and a man's head fly one way and his feet the other. On this first attack, a Co. I's aids man was killed by a sniper and another was wounded in the leg, so just as on April 14th and 15th there was plenty of work for the Aid man that was left. It seems as though I always get into those situations. Ha! Ha! In those hours before dawn, a sniper got our Commanding Officer right between the eyes, dead instantly. That was really some "initiation" we got as to what combat was like. But I lived and that's what counts, doesn't it???? I'll continue starting at dawn Tuesday, Feb. 20th, okay???

I see by your letter on May 5th that you also received that parcel that I sent from Florence containing those gifts. Are you sure you enjoyed them as much as you say you do?? I'm afraid my wife is disappointed because she didn't get any cameras but those that looked half decent cost an exorbitant fee and I wasn't that well stocked in funds. Even so, you probably have no idea what the things cost that I did get you and the folks. They really should be good, believe me!!!!! I'm sorry to hear that one of those beads had fallen out. Can't you fix it???? Maybe I can get some other things if I'm able to get to a place, but things are so exorbitantly high in price.

Do you think I'd be sorry I married you because you think you do a lot of complaining?? I'd be very disappointed if my Honey wouldn't tell me every time that she doesn't feel well. That is an order and I surely don't think she's complaining

when she tells me how she feels. How is your cold anyway??
I hope it's all gone by this time!! Did those pills help you???
Honestly, I'm sure that no man could possibly have received a
finer wife than I have. My, but I'm lucky!!!

Say, Flush really must be growing and developing into a
very cute dog. I'm anxious to see her. How is Judy??? Is she
still jealous of Flush??

O but I love you so very much and I guess I'm affected
the same way you are when I think of coming home. It,
"thrills" me all to pieces. Why are you so good to me?? Gosh,
but you're the Dearest Wife in all the world.

[Wednesday] May 30th

Well, today is Memorial Day or Decoration Day as many
people term it. This is another holiday I'm not spending with
those I love and gosh that hurts. This morning from 8 to
10:30 we had a road march and at 11 AM the whole 3rd
Battalion paid tribute to those who gave their "lives" in our
World War. We all stood attention and then the playing of
taps. It was a very, very impressive service. Yes, we have
won the war in Europe, but we paid a very "Dear" price in
human lives. Let's hope that peace will come quickly in the
Pacific and that out of it all, we get enduring peace for all
time.

Yesterday we left our area at about 6 AM but didn't hit
Venice until about 10:15. We made connections at Udine
with a "convoy" and the convoy was late so that's why it took
us over 4 hours. That city is worth seeing. It's so big that you
couldn't see nearly all of it in the short time we had but they
showed us the main points of interest. Those canals and
gondolas are really what struck me. Everything you read
about and saw pictures of concerning these canals is correct.
You can't get around unless you take a gondola. The main

street is about the width of Penn St. and it's, of course, a canal, known as the Grand Canal. Practically every house a boat and then at every square, they have lots of gondolas sitting just as we have taxi stands in our cities. The canals range in width from small alleys up to this big grand canal and gosh but it's interesting to see all these boats pass each other coming out from one canal to another just like street intersections in our cities and hardly ever as much as touch each other. Among the most interesting sights we saw was the famous Cathedral of St. Marco[95], St. Marco Square, the huge tower in the square[96] you can walk up to the top of for 10 cents or ride up in an elevator for 15 cents. Well, I naturally chose to ride. Ha! Ha! The view was wonderful. At 2:30 PM they took us to a movie. The picture was "The Road to Frisco" starring George Raft, Ann Sheridan, and Humphrey Bogart. It was quite an old picture but I can't remember ever seeing it. You eat in mess halls similar to the one we had in Florence and the meal does not cost you a single penny. I managed to sit right at the window and look right out onto the canal. I certainly did enjoy myself and I think my wife and I will have to come over to Venice after the war and spend about a month there.

In Venice, I met a fellow I knew from Barkeley. He was also in the Second Battalion and knew Ed quite well. I realize my Darling, how difficult it must be to write to his girlfriend. I don't know if I should write, or not? He wrote to his parents and girlfriend so much about me and he told me that they all

---

[95] Better known as Saint Mark's Basilica, located in the Piazza San Marco, it was consecrated in 1117.

[96] St. Marks Campanile is the bell tower of St. Marks Basilica. It is 323 feet tall with a pyramid shaped spire. It has been restored several times over the decades with a complete collapse in 1902, reopening in 1912-1000 years after its original foundation was laid.

felt as though they knew me. He'd always show me the part of the letters in which they referred to me. I feel so sorry for them. This fellow told me that his only brother who is in the Air Corps had been missing in action but they just heard that he had been taken prisoner of war. Now they have to get the news that Ed was killed. Too bad!!!!!

Dearest, coming back now to those pictures you had taken and you're even sending me one of the big ones. It seems that $24.00 is a lot of money to spend on pictures but yet, they are something you'll always have and believe me, I think they are such very good pictures. The folder in which you sent the picture just fits in my pocket nicely and goes wherever I go. It's always with me, always, so don't think that I'm scaring the rats with it because in the first place we don't have any rats out here and in the second place it's such a wonderful picture that I'm sure it couldn't scare anyone. Ha! Ha!

What is the world are those Allentown and Reading Transit people striking for?? Gosh, but the transportation systems are having trouble with their employees. Yes, I remember very well how we used to use those Temple buses and how we complained sometimes of the inconvenience. Well, when we are all united again, I'm sure we'll appreciate everything in life to a far greater degree than we did in the past.

[Thursday] May 31st

My time is limited but I'll have to find time to at least write a V Mail. Will my Honey Bunch forgive me?? This morning they took us down to the shower unit. We were also waiting in line to have our teeth checked when a "shower" came up and so that was postponed to a later date.

[Friday] June 1st

This morning we had a parade in which our whole 85th Regiment took part and also some attached units. The parade took place about 5 miles from where we are situated. Some Regimental Officers and enlisted men received decorations but here is something that is news. Our Battalion was, I believe, the first one to arrive at the parade grounds and as we were marching into our preliminary positions there was a group of "musicians" to our right and guess who was standing there with a trombone in his hand but "William"!! Gosh, but I was surprised. I was supposed to be marching at attention but even so, I left out a "Yello". He saw me and laughed too but I couldn't get out of rank. He played with the band during the parade and after it was over, I so much wanted to see him but we were rushed away in our trucks immediately after it was over. That was the first fellow I really knew quite well and then I couldn't even get to talk to him.

After dinner, I wanted to immediately start writing to my Sweet Wife but then I discovered that Headquarters Co. was scheduled to play Medics in softball and here they demanded that I umpire the game. I couldn't refuse because it was an order from my superiors!!! Well, I umpired and you guessed it, this time the Medics won 9-5. You see today they had the umpire on their side. Ha! Ha!

Well, the rumor has it again that we're moving tomorrow morning, they say into a small town very near here. Here's something that my Dearest might not like. The rumor also says that we'll be in this immediate area for about four or five months. Well, it could be a lot worse for we could be leaving for the Pacific at this moment.

I guess I'll continue my experience from where I left off. Well, our Battalion held Belvedere against a couple of German counterattacks and while most of our casualties came during that dawn attack, we still encountered some trouble but all counterattacks were beaten off. Not only did I administer first aid but they were so short of litter bearers that we had to pitch in and help evacuate. Yes, I was going all that day and my, oh my, I was tired that night. That afternoon our Company (Co. I) moved off Belvedere to a neighboring slope and relieved a Company from the First Battalion. That was Feb 20th. Honestly, I really experienced some sights. It's terrible how war ruins so many, many lives. Those first three days cost our one Company over 50 of their men. When you come to think of it one can hardly believe that such things must be. We remained on this particular ridge until the night of Feb 27th (Tuesday night). On Sunday night a patrol went out from this ridge and ran into some trouble from enemy machine gun and mortar fire. We had two rather serious casualties but both the men lived. One had his foot blown off. Gosh, I hate those night patrols because you'll never know when you'll run into some "Jerry" fire. They can usually see you but you can't see them. On Tuesday night about midnight, a unit from the Brazilian Expeditionary Force[97] relieved us and we moved back about 2000 yards to another ridge where we still received quite a bit of artillery fire but no mortar fire. We stayed there until the early morning of March 3rd (Saturday). I'll stop here and continue in a later letter.

So, William was in the hospital for a few days. William never seemed very strong and I can easily see how his nerves would get the best of him if the 86th had any experiences that the 85th had. This morning when I saw him, he seemed to have a very "full" face and looked very well. Maybe he's been reassigned to the band now or probably it was just a job for today.

---

[97] Brazil sent ground troop support into the war in Italy from 1944-1945.

You tell Charlie that I asked about him and that in 1948 he won't be able to vote Roosevelt but he shouldn't worry, the Democrats will have another good man on the ticket and he'll sweep the country. (I hope). Ha! Ha! Charlie, you know is a very hard Republican. Ha! Ha!

I heard some remark too, about Camp Barkeley closing down, evidently, it must be true if Stan said so also. Yes, I bet Abilene is a regular "ghost" town once all those soldiers leave. We certainly did have a wonderful time down in Texas, didn't we???

No, my Dearest, I still haven't gotten those Hershey bars!![98] Did you send in a request to the Hershey plant or just how did you go about ordering then??? I too, can't see how they are delayed for such a long time.

Yes, my Dearest, I'm positively certain that there isn't another soldier who writes as many letters as I do, at least to my Dear Wife and Parents. Gosh, some fellows don't write to their people for weeks at a time. Of course, nobody receives as much mail as I do either, so that equals everything. I'm the luckiest soldier in the U.S. Army.

Gosh, alive you and Sister were rough on Mother and Grandma on Mother's Day. You won four straight games from them!! Mother writes and tells me you and Sister "cheat".

[Saturday] June 2nd
Darling Sugar Plum,

How does my Sweetheart like that for a salutation??? Ha! Ha! Well, no matter what I greet her with she is absolutely the Dearest in all the world and I love her so very much. No

---

[98] From 1941 through 1945 Hershey produced more than a billion ration bars for the troops. They introduced some different chocolates in the mid 1900's which included Mr. Goodbar, Krackel, Minatures and Kisses.

mail from anyone thus far today!! It seems as though we're getting our mail either noon or rather late in the evening. So, we'll probably have mail call tonight. I certainly hope so because I'm anxious to receive mail.

This morning at about 8:05 we went on another road march and gee-whiz our M.A.C. Officer, who led the road march, got lost and we barely got back for our noon meal. We haven't hiked that far at the pace we traveled since our march through the Po Valley.

I guess I'll continue some more of my experiences while over here in Italy. Well, it was 7 AM on March 3rd after a half-hour of artillery barrage that we shoved off again from this ridge we were occupying. Our opposition wasn't so very strong. Oh, we had quite a few casualties but nothing like we experienced on Belvedere. We had a few Medics wounded but none killed. On those three days on Belvedere and the surrounding ridges, we lost 14 men out of 38 in our Medical Station. That included killed and wounded. Well, on March 3rd we took quite a few additional ridges and rounded up many German prisoners. On Sunday too we were quite busy because I'm quite sure I wasn't able to write on either the 4th or the 3rd. Well, we were able to sleep in a building, just a very few of us, from the 3rd of March until Thursday night, March 8th. At about midnight we moved out of those positions and walked for about 3 hours until Friday the 9th when we stopped and they told us to "dig" in for the night. Well, I only got about 3 hours of sleep that night. In the morning they told us that we were going to get showers so at about 9 AM we walked to the nearest road (Highway 63) where trucks could pick us up and take us back about 10 miles to a "mobile" shower unit. We remained at this same position Friday night and until March 11th. We were gotten up and again walked to the Highway where a huge truck convoy was waiting for us and we were transported back to that city where we had those few days of rest. The town they took us to was Montecatini. It was a very nice town, by far the largest we had ever been in and it contained a nice Red Cross building too. The building contained a courtyard in the center and around the courtyard they had ping pong tables. At one end of the yard, the building contained a huge auditorium where movies and USO stage shows were held. We arrived in this town at about 8 AM on Sunday (11th). After chow, I ran all over town to locate Protestant Services and finally found out they were held right in the auditorium in the Red Cross building. Well, we remained in this town until Wednesday morning (March 14th) at 10 AM when we took off again for the front lines. Yes, those three days we spent there were really a vacation. We ate good meals, slept on cots in buildings, and could write letters at desks amid pleasant surroundings. That was the life. Ha! Ha! Well, I'll let my story end again on March 14th, is that alright???

Now, my Sweetheart, you absolutely must not worry about me having enough money. I have plenty of money, have no fear. That's right, I believe I forgot to mention it but we got paid on Thursday. I got my usual salary of $17.25 again so you can see I have plenty of money. Ha! Ha!

I must laugh at your letter of May 15th; my Dear hadn't planned to go up home but when she heard that in the evening mail they received two letters, she immediately got the Chevy and went up. So, my Darling held a $500 bill in your hand!! Yes, those are quite nice things to have in your hand and to really own. I've held them in my hands many times when I worked in the post office. Of course, they weren't mine. Ha! Ha! Daddy got a good price for Howard's car!! Automobiles fetch a fancy price these days, don't they???

We have a new M.A.C. officer. Lt. Liotta was our original M.A.C. officer but he was moved to a collecting company. Nevin is still our M.C. officer. Yes, all our M.C. officers are doctors. Nevin was a Doctor in a New York hospital before entering the service.

Dearest, you mustn't worry in the least about these Italian girls. I see very few of them because I don't look for them and the ones I do see, are certainly nothing on the eyes. No woman can beat my honey for "looks".

[Sunday] June 3rd

This morning at 8 AM we had worship services as usual. I attended. The chaplain had a fine service; his theme was "Christ and Human Weakness". At 10 AM we had a Battalion formation by the highway. We received a visitor who reviewed our troops, and guess who it was, none other than General R.L.G. Alexander, Commander-in-Chief of all Allied Forces in the Mediterranean Theater of Operations. Yes, and I saw him too. Alexander is a big man, so I feel rather honored to have been able to see him.

After an early chow, we got our equipment ready and moved into a nearby town. There is fixing up to be done, I don't think the setup will be too bad. I can sleep on a "litter" and managed to get a mattress over it so it is pretty comfortable. The latest rumor has us moving on Tuesday and quite a distance too. I wish they'd make up their mind. Ha! Ha!

[Monday] June 4th

There are six of us sleeping in one room and all but one has managed to "rig" up something to sleep on. He, of course, is sleeping on the floor, which is still a lot better than sleeping outside. This afternoon our 3rd Battalion Medics are going to play the 2nd Battalion Medics in softball and I've again been elected to umpire. We must stand reveille at 6:30 and retreat at 5 PM every day.

I'll again continue my experiences in Italy. I don't think our letters are censored anymore so I can write practically anything I please. At 10 AM Wednesday, we loaded trucks and they took us back toward the front lines. At about 4 PM we disembarked and walked for about 2 hours, then told to "dig in". This area was subject to artillery fire. We stayed here Wed and Thursday until 7 PM. We were scheduled to relieve a company of the 1st Battalion (Co. C) which had taken this ridge and were suffering quite a few casualties in holding it from mortar and artillery fire. Every Battalion is divided into companies plus a Headquarters Co. The 1st Battalion is made up of Co.'s A, B, C, & D; the 2nd Battalion is made up of Co.'s E, F, G & H, and the 3rd Battalion is made up of Co.'s I, K, L & M. Ed was attached to Co. E, 2nd Battalion, and Norman was in Co. C, 1st Battalion. We relieved Co. C that Thursday night (March 15th) and it was on this ridge about three days before that Norman was killed. It was "hell" there. Those "krauts" had that hill "zeroed" to a tee. We lost a few men too while there and quite a few wounded. So, I know exactly where and how Norman was killed. I was lucky enough to be in a building again on this ridge where the Commanding Officer of Co. I had his C.P. but gosh that building was almost more hazardous than a fox hole because the Germans had perfect vision on it and landing shells all around it day and night. A day or so after we left there, they made a Direct Hit on the house. We remained on this ridge until Wednesday morning (March 28th) at 3:30 AM. It was here that I constantly pulled phone guard. We have phones "rigged up" right on the front lines. You see, the medic had to be ready to treat wounded all hours of the day and night and if a shell would hit anyone they'd call up and we'd rush to that point. I'll continue from this point in a later letter.

[Tuesday] June 5th

Now don't faint when I tell you this. Ha! Ha! Yesterday I received twelve (12) letters from home. Eight of them were from the folks up home and four from my Darling Wife. Then this afternoon right before the evening meal I found four more letters on my bed, two from my Sweetheart and two from the folks at home which made sixteen letters in two days. I knew I was missing a lot.

This afternoon we had a softball game between two teams from our own medics. That's right I again was the umpire. Ha! Ha! The way it looks I'll be a professional umpire before the war is over. This town we are staying in is called Cividale[99] and it is about 100 miles Northwest of Venice.

Guess I'll continue some more of my experiences. You seem to enjoy reading them but if you are going to let it worry you maybe I'd better discontinue them. How about it??? I might add that on Sunday, March 18th, we had church services in an old barn that had been shelled unmercifully by our troops in driving out the Germans. We also spent Palm Sunday at this same place but I couldn't for the life of me find out when or where Protestant services were held. So that day I worshiped by myself which isn't bad at all. Well, on Wednesday morning (March 28th) a company from the 2nd Battalion relieved us and during those early morning hours, we hiked back to the place we had disembarked from the trucks that brought us from Montecatini on Wed. March 14th.

---

[99] The name of this town is actually Cividale del Friuli, situated at the foothills of the Eastern Alps. It's medieval history dates back before 50 B.C. with the Roman Empire.

Gosh, and that was some hike!! It was raining and muddy and it was up and down all the time. Down one Mt. slope and up another and so on, and I really had a heavy pack on my back, too. But you know your hubby is pretty "tough". Ha! Ha! I guess a fellow can take almost anything!!!! We were again met by trucks and guess where we went--back to Prunetta, the same place we had been twice before. That town seemed to be the town where the 3rd Battalion of our Regiment always reorganized and re-equipped itself for its next assignment. Well, about 4:30 Wed afternoon, after I had gotten things pretty well settled at our place in Prunetta I was told that in the morning I would start for Florence. I'll continue my story as of March 29th in a later letter.

My Dear, I can just taste that good bologna even though it is only on the way over to me. I just know that it will be very, very good.

[Wednesday] June 6th

My Dearest Peachy,

I love peaches very much and you are no exception. Ha! Ha! You know since we moved into buildings the days have been very lovely, but practically the whole time we were living in pup tents we had rain. Isn't it strange the way those things happen???

This morning we had to put up our mosquito nets over our bunks. We have to arrange these nets so that when you are in bed the net will completely enclose you. I understand that the anopheles mosquito gets around these parts and there are a few cases of malaria so we have to take the necessary precautions. They say that parts of the Po Valley are malaria-infested. You must always be on the "alert" for something. Ha! Ha!

This afternoon the 3rd Battalion Medics played the 1st Battalion Medics in softball. The 1st Battalion is about 27 miles from here and the game didn't get started until 3 PM. They also had an umpire so we had an umpire for the bases and one behind the plate. We had a rather bad day for our team lost by the convincing score of 18-2.

I don't believe I mentioned this but on Monday night we were put on a three-day alert; that is any time in those next three days we had to be ready to move out on a three-hour notice. We were told that Marshal Tito[100] was moving about 5,000 of his men and if necessary, we would move too. However, I was told that the "alert" was called off.

Here goes again on some of my experiences. Well, at 9 AM (Thursday, March 29th) our Medical truck took me to a town called Campo Tizzaro, which was about 15 to 20 miles. We arrived there at about 10 AM. This town was the Headquarters for our 85th Regiment and all the Medics who were on a pass from all Battalions came here. The rest of the morning we were given orientation as to how these passes would work, how long they'd be, what the uniform would be, and the like. All the men from the whole Regiment came here to this town and we were only going to leave for Florence the following morning. The rest of the afternoon I walked around the town. I had wanted to take a shower but the line was much too long. That evening I went to a barber and got my hair cut. Thursday night we were issued cots and would have slept in what was formerly a garage, but a couple of fellows whom I knew slightly asked me to go with them, that they found a private home for four fellows. The people they said were very nice and they had beds with "clean white sheets" to

---

[100] Marshal Tito was the leader of the Yugoslavian Communist Partisans and during this time there was a Post War border dispute between Italy and Yugoslavia that was peacefully solved.

sleep on. That sounded too good to be true so I went along and gosh the people were very nice and the place was so clean too. That mattress certainly did feel very good and they also let me write my two mails of March 29th at the kitchen table. It was a middle-aged couple with a daughter about 5 or 6 years old. I'll leave now and continue from this point later.

No, my Sweetheart, I don't think the Italians play baseball, in fact, I haven't seen or heard any sport which they partake in. I'm sure they aren't the sports-loving people we Americans are.

[Thursday] June 7th

Starting at 9:00 this morning until 4:00 this afternoon I've been giving "shots". By that I mean we injected for typhoid, tetanus, and smallpox. I and another fellow were giving the tetanus injections. Soon, we'll also give "typhus" injections. I'm getting to be an "artist" at the trade. Some of the older men in the outfit who are supposed to know the stuff absolutely don't know what the "score" is. I laugh; the men try and get in line so that I give them their shots rather than the Sergeant who was "shooting" with me. These guys have been in the "Medics" for two, three years, and still don't know their job.

Here goes again on some of my experiences. We left on March 30th around 8 AM heading for Florence. We reported at 1 PM to be checked in to receive our admission cards which would entitle us to all our meals and any entertainments which might be held, such as USO shows, movies, and the like. The building we stayed which used to be a railroad terminal was huge and magnificent. The mess hall where we ate was formally the railroad restaurant and it was immense. The Red Cross room was formally the huge lobby of the railroad station. The 2nd and 3rd floors were

probably all offices in normal times but now all the rooms
had cots in them with mattresses on them. I had a very
enjoyable stay in Florence. It was wonderful just to take your
good old time in doing everything. We left Florence at about
2:00 on Tuesday, April 3rd. I'll continue in a later letter.

Dearest, that is a very fine idea which your parents have
about you getting a bicycle and taking rides with them
because when I get home, I'll either get mine fixed or buy
another one and all four of us will go riding.

[Friday] June 8th

What a hot day this has been!!! As I'm writing this letter
the perspiration is just pouring down my arms and forehead.
This morning we had an hour of class drill and following that
we went on a two-hour road march and "whew" this Italian
sun is really hot!!!! This afternoon we saw a movie entitled
"On To Tokyo".[101] It was a film explaining what soldiers
would go to the Pacific, how they would go, and the like. It
said what I already had heard that most of the combat troops
that would go to the Pacific would go by way of the States
and receive a furlough. Whether that will happen or not I
guess nobody knows.

[Saturday] June 9th

Well, today is the big day at Churchill Downs in
Kentucky, the annual running of the Kentucky Derby.[102]
Remember, my Sweet, how I picked the winner last year,

---

[101] This was a propagandistic type short documentary designed to
enlighten the American citizens about how the war might end in Japan. It
showed the destruction of war both by the allies and the enemy, battles at
Guam and the Air Force capacity on Saipan getting prepared to bomb
Japan.
[102] This was the 71st Kentucky Derby with Hoop Jr. winning and Pot of
Luck coming in second.

Pensive, you know was my choice. I haven't been able to keep up with the horses this year so I wouldn't attempt to name the winner. Ha! Ha!

Last night I received a box from My Honey. Don't send any more chocolate candy because they were quite soft; the Tootsie Rolls were in very good shape.

I'll continue now on my doings. After four days in Florence, we arrived at our Regimental Medical Depot at about 6:30 PM and arrived at our Battalion Aid Station around 9 PM. You see on Easter Sunday, April 1st our battalion again left Prunetta and came back to the front and again took up "holding" positions a little to the west of where we had been before going to Prunetta. That Tuesday night I read my mail until midnight. The next morning (April 4th) I went back to my Company. Most of the men were living in fox holes, but once again I was very fortunate and lived in some sort of barn having straw as my bed. I'll continue here in a later letter. Okay???

I resent that question you asked me about being "afraid" to fly home!!! I can't think of a thing anymore short of war itself that would make me afraid. Ha! Ha! I certainly would not be afraid to fly home knowing who was waiting for me when I reached my destination. No, my Dear, I do not keep a diary. All the dates stick with a fellow pretty well. I'm sure that some of them I'll never forget. You bet, my Sweetheart, we'll make up for all these lonely days we've spent apart from each other. We must thank "God" many, many times for looking after me the way he did.

I've mentioned in a previous letter, on Belvedere there were well over 50% of the men in Co. I, either wounded or killed. I'd say that about 75% of the casualties on Belvedere were wounded and 25% were killed. I also mentioned the 14th and 15th of April we lost about 150 to 155 men out of a company whose strength was around 200. In other words, 75% or better were casualties. The % killed here was greater than on Belvedere but still, there were more wounded than killed. I'd say about 60% wounded and 40 % killed. Yes, we were "slaughtered" those two days. Honey, there are close to 1500 men in a Battalion including "attached" units. There are 38 Medics attached to a Battalion, 12 Company Aid men, 18 Evacuation men, and 8 men who work in the Aid Station. There are about 4500 men in the 85th Regiment and anywhere from 12,500 to 15,000 men in the 10th Mt. Division.

[Sunday] June 10th

My Honey, your letters were so interesting but you shouldn't have let the fact that I received the "Bronze Star" make you so nervous and jumpy. Ha! Ha! Your hubby is still the same man whom you waved goodbye to at the station on Nov. 29th. No matter what he has, he's still the same man, and don't you go and think I'm so wonderful all of a sudden. Naturally, it's something that you're glad to have but believe me, I'm not sticking out my chest now, I'm just thankful I'm alive to wear it. One of our Medics who was killed was awarded the Bronze Star posthumously. I felt sorry, especially since he had three children, but such is war. I'll get around someday to tell you what happened on the 15th of April but what little I've told you so far you seem to be overcome with "chills" so I better stop telling you such things. No, not all the medics got those "Medals". It makes a fellow feel good though when he can save a man's life rather than "take" it.

Last night I was C.Q. (Charge of Quarters) at the Aide Station. Every night there is someone who stays at the Aid Station in case someone comes in for any first aid or any medicine. They have a cot in the Aid Station and the C.Q. sleeps right there. If during the night anyone takes sick suddenly, they contact you by phone and you, in turn, send the ambulance after them. Fellows came in during the evening with burns, athlete's foot, and diarrhea. So, I was not too busy.

This morning we had church services in an Italian movie house in town. There were very many soldiers there too. I'm usually the only Medic going to church but four other fellows asked me this morning if I'd mind if they'd go with me. One of the fellows (he just joined our outfit about May 1st) who had been at a Replacement Depot for some time and had been overseas for two years said that this was only the third church service he'd been at since he's in the Army and the first two were attended while he was still in the States. I can't see how a fellow can "live" without attending church especially at times such as these.

Today I'm sure is Father's Day and again I want to wish our Father's the best in everything and the hope that they will be in some way rewarded for all the things they have done for us. Gee whiz, I only wish I could spend the day with them but believe me I'm with them in mind and spirit and by this time next year, we'll celebrate the day together. How about it??? What did you get our Father's anyway?? Be sure and "jot down" how much it all costs because I'm certainly going to pay for all of it. Now that's an order from your "boss" and he means it too. Ha! Ha!

Honey, you asked me how I found out about "Ed"?? I found out through our Mail Clerk who gets the mail for all the medics in our Regiment. I found out on the 27th of April when he casually mentioned the names of the medics who had been killed up to that time. Gosh, it struck me hard when I first heard that. He and I were such great friends and the day he was killed I don't believe I was more than 1000 yds. away from him. We were on neighboring ridges.

Honey Bunch, we just had mail call and I was lucky again, I received three V-Mails from my Darling Wife and was so sorry to hear that my Sweetheart was troubled by a small dent in the fender. Why did you cry over such a little thing?? Dearest, that happens to anybody, and don't think for one minute that I'm angry or troubled by such a small thing. Now please, please don't worry about such small things and don't think now that you must get it fixed just for me. I'm not coming home to see the car but to see my folks and my Dearest Darling Wife. I really should bawl you out for taking such a thing so seriously. Ha! Ha! When we have our lives, what is there to worry about?? Nothing!!! I've got dents in the fenders plenty of times and everyone else does too.

[Monday] June 11th

Here we go on another week and we're still in the town of Cividale and we'll be here for some time the way things appear to me. Darling, you just watch those two St. Louis teams. They're climbing all the time and before you know it, they'll be in first place.

[Tuesday] June 12th

Last night we got our PX rations in and it took quite a few hours to break it all down and have every man get his. My rations cost $3.20 which included candy, cookies, beer, cigarettes, soap, and the like. I sold my beer and cigarettes to some other fellow but the rest I kept. This morning we chanced off some more ration things and I received an airmail tablet-price 15 cents. After that twelve of us got our truck and went for showers.

I guess I'll continue some more of my experiences although I honestly believe you'd rather not hear them. It worries you too much and I can't see why because I'm O.K. and well so why worry? I believe I left off on the morning of April 4th. We only remained on this ridge until Friday, April 6th. We moved out about 4 PM about a mile to our "rear" assembly area. We medics stayed in a building there. Here we learned all about the big push that was going to come off the following week, what day we didn't know. We remained here until Saturday morning, April 14th at 9 AM, when we took off on our push. From Monday the 9th until the day we left we were given various orientations as to what was coming off. I knew then that it was going to be "rugged" especially the first days. Our 3rd Battalion had by far the toughest deal in our Regiment and we all realized it too. On Wednesday at noon (April 11th) we were told the "it" was coming off the next morning but at 6:30 PM that night it was called off and postponed for twenty-four hours because the weather bureau predicted cloudy weather the next morning and our planes could not operate as efficiently in cloudy weather. You see we were going to have quite a lot of air support. Well, we had rain on Thursday and although it cleared about 5 PM, they again postponed it another 24 hours this time because the roads and fields were pretty muddy and our "tanks" would not be able to operate to as great an efficiency point as if they would with dry "footing". Everything had to be just right because they knew that it all had to be coordinated or the results might be negative and there were too many boy's lives at stake. Friday morning, the 13th, we heard about Roosevelt's death and I just couldn't believe it. Gee but that struck me hard. I couldn't help but feel that it struck all of you pretty hard too. It shocked the whole country. I'll continue here in a later letter.

As of May 12th, I had 29 points; 10 months of service in the Army-10 points, 4 months overseas service 4 points, two Battle Participation Stars-10 points, and my Bronze Star Medal- 5 points or a total of 29 points. Yes, my Sweetheart, triplets would have given us 65 points but it certainly would have helped. Ha! Ha! We are really going to "make the dust fly". How about it?? They are trying to get us another Battle Star for crossing Lake la Garda but I'm not sure if we'll get it or not. That would give me 15 more points. It's not very many points but think of the fellows who are just entering the service. They are starting with "zero" unless they have children. Darling, I think it wouldn't be a bad idea at all to see the Doctor again. I feel sure that there is nothing wrong with either of us but it wouldn't do any harm just to get a checkup. Our "time" will come, have no fear, my Sweetheart!!!

[Wednesday] June 13th

This morning we had an hour of Close Order Drill after which we had two hours of orientation on the Far East situation. You know there are very few days that I've missed writing but I enjoy it so much because it brings me closer to home and I enjoy thinking of the enjoyable times that the future holds for all of us.

Well, I'll continue again with my experiences. At 9 AM we took off for our Assembly area. I had joined Co. I earlier that morning and received final instructions from the Company Commander as to what the objective of Co. I would be. We, together with Co. K were going to spearhead the 3rd Battalions attack and Co. L was going to remain in reserve. From 8:30 to 9 AM we had an artillery barrage that rocked the "universe". Ha! Ha! Gosh, I couldn't see how anyone could have survived that "barrage" but they did because they gave us plenty of trouble those next two days. At exactly 9

AM we started. We walked over a few ridges and at about 10 AM they started landing in their artillery and mortars. At the moment we (Co. I) were on a steep ridge on a reverse slope and the artillery was hitting us too much. They were hitting on the forward slope but the "shrapnel" was flying around all about us. When the head of our Company took off over the top of the ridge, the "Krauts" opened up with machine-gun fire. They had the whole top of the ridge "zeroed" and whenever a fellow took off over the top, they'd "mow" him down with machine-gun fire. Well, I had "lots of business" right there. I'd pull or drag the wounded from the top of the ridge over on the reverse slope but the "bastards" even fired upon me anyway. The "bums" didn't respect the Red Cross I had painted on my helmet. After our company was pinned down on this slope, until the middle of the afternoon when a few men broke through and wiped out the German machine-gun nests with hand grenades, we finally moved off the slope. We wiped out some more enemy installations but again late that afternoon, after suffering so many casualties, we retreated to the slope we had been pinned down on and we were told to dig in for the night. We had not reached our objective which they had planned to have us reach by the end of that day because resistance was too heavy. So, they said that tomorrow we had to push off again. One trouble was that a couple of Companies in the second Battalion (one of which was Ed's Co.) were supposed to take the ridges on our "right flank" but they didn't keep up with us and as a result, we were exposed on our left and right flank as well as to our front and they were spraying us with machine-gun fire unmercifully. The sights I saw that day were horrible. On top of it, all the Germans had cleverly laid minefields which "took" a lot of our men. One of our platoons walked "plum" into a minefield and suffered heavily. How I ever managed not to step on any is a miracle. One had to "hug" the ground constantly so that you would not expose yourself to machine-gun fire and yet be careful not to hit a mine. I'll continue from here in a later letter. I won't tell you all my experiences these few days because you'll become too "jumpy". When I get home, I'll relate it all.

So, William is in "Riva". Well, that town is very familiar to me because we too were in that town. We were there when the war in Italy was declared officially over. The town is along Lake La Garda, the upper end of the Lake. The scenery is really beautiful. We were there from Tues, May 1st until Sat May 5th. Yesterday, our Sgt. asked how many men would like to play in a band orchestra and one other fellow and I submitted our names. Glad to hear Donald is situated so close to home. I hope he'll be alright. Do they plan to remove the shrapnel from his side?? What outfit is Eugene attached to since he's coming home shortly???

Honey Bunch, did you get your watch repaired?? I hope too that it will work well this time. I know one thing that I'm going to buy my Honey when I get home even though she wants a "ring" in the bargain. She can have both the ring and the watch, that's how much I love my Darling.

That fellow Leroy who taught for Otis that one Sunday he left early is a very nice chap. He hasn't attended our Sunday School very long. He belongs to Zion's Church, I think but attends our Sunday School now.

[Thursday] June 14th

There's a rumor circulating this evening that we're going to have a two-day problem tomorrow and Saturday. What kind of problem it will be I don't know?

Honey Darling, you seem to worry a lot about that bill you owe at the garage. I'm sure Warren and Allen aren't worried about it as much as you are. They don't mind because they know they will get their money sooner or later.

Honey Bunch, as you probably know I'm still in the town of Cividale and it is only about 90 miles from Trieste. No, we are not too far from Austria and Yugoslavia. Rumors have it we will go to Austria before long.

[Saturday] June 16th

Late last night I had the good fortune of receiving another box from my Sweetheart and gosh, was I glad to get what was in it!! One Lebanon Bologna[103], 1 box of Potato Sticks, one can of fruit salad, and a can of Nestles' Cocoa. I started on the bologna before I went to bed and ate some more of it this morning. Thank you for being so considerate. That bologna really must have cost you not only a lot of money but also quite a few points.

This morning we had an hour of close-order drill, followed by an inspection of our building and "ourselves". Next Tuesday we have a "problem" that is a "dry run" of actual combat conditions. At 11 AM today we were oriented as to what it would be like. It will last only from 6 in the morning until 3 in the afternoon.

Would you like to hear more about my experiences?? If you insist, I'll tell you a few more. I stopped on the evening of April 14th. After treating casualties that night until about 11 PM, I started digging my fox hole. I was quite tired but it is amazing how much energy a fellow possesses when that artillery and mortar fire is landing all about you. At dawn (April 15th) we again set out and that day I'm sure I'll never forget. The Commanding Officer told us that we had to take

---

[103] This is cured, smoked and fermented sausage made from beef, which was developed in the 19th Century by the Pennsylvania Dutch of Lebanon County, Pa.

our objective at all costs. That whole day was spent capturing and mopping up our scheduled ridges which were the "key" points in opening up our way into the Po Valley. Well, we got all we were supposed to get but it "cost" us heavily. Advancing against point-blank machine-gun fire with mortar and artillery shells dropping all the time is no picnic. Ha! Ha! Ha! To have fellows blown to bits twenty feet from you and not get much yourself is a miracle. We dug in once for a few hours and a mortar made a direct hit on the fox hole right above mine in which there were three fellows. It is needless to say what the results were. You might want to know what I did to have received the Bronze Star. I'm afraid it would sound too fantastic if I were to write it and I'm sure you wouldn't feel good about it. When I was told back around the beginning of May that I was put in for a "citation" I thought it was a lot of "baloney" but the order actually did come through. I had been put in for Belvedere too but as yet nothing has happened about that. "Doc" Nevin said that a recommendation for the "Silver Star" had been put in for me on this last push, but that also has not come through as yet. I told him I was only doing my duty, so please don't go thinking you have such a heroic husband. He's the same fellow you married back in 1939. Ha! Ha! Ha! I'll continue more of my tales later.

So, Aunt Sally will make some more fudge for me!! That candy is the best you can find. Darling, you shouldn't have cleaned and waxed the car on Memorial Day when it was so cold. Gosh, I bet your fingers were cold. My Honey Bunch takes excellent care of the car and please don't think that I think any less of your driving because you got a dent in it.

There are only two fellows in a pup tent. This fellow I pitched with is a few years younger than I am. He's been in the Army for three years now.

Darling, you asked me about the Italian girls!! I don't know too much about them except what I see of them walking the streets. On the whole, I'd say they look just about the same as the average American girl. They dress about the same except that their shoes are funny-looking wooden contraptions. You hardly ever see them wearing stockings and they say that a pair of stockings run anywhere from $10 to $50, so I guess there's a reason for them not wearing them. Very few people over here can speak English. You meet a few who have picked up a little here and there.

[Sunday] June 17th

My Dearest Heart Throb,

My heart always beats at a fast tempo when I think of my Sweetheart. According to your letters, today is Father's Day and I thought it was last Sunday. No letters for me yesterday and of course none today as yet but last night I received two copies of the Ursinus News.

This morning we had Sunday services in the Italian movie house. Gosh, but there were lots of soldiers present. I bet it was the best-attended service we've had since we left the states. The chaplain's theme for his sermon was "The Road Back". For the rest of the morning, I read the "Stars & Stripes". Immediately after the noon meal, I started your letter. Most of the fellows are in town and it is nice and quiet.

Well here goes again on some more of my happenings. As I said April 15th was probably the "worst" day in my Army "career". That whole night the Germans continued throwing in mortars and artillery plus attempting several counter-attacks but in each case were driven back. When dawn came Monday morning, we could see by the dead scattered about how expensive war is on human lives; many men whom I knew and lived with and talked to daily. About noon we moved to another ridge and 1/2 a mile from where we were, dug in. This ridge had been taken by the 2nd Battalion and we relieved them. That night we were supposed to be relieved by the Brazilians but they never did come. That night only a few artillery shells came in and nobody in our company was hurt. Tuesday we just maintained our position until about 10 PM when the Brazilians relieved us. We descended to the highway below until all the companies in the Battalion had been relieved. Then, company by company, in a single file we took off down the highway. We walked for about two hours and then took off on some side road and each company took a field and we "dug in" again. Wednesday morning, we were again ordered to hit the road and we walked and walked and walked. We reached our destination at about 6:30 PM Wednesday. Gee whiz, all I did for about an hour after that was treat sore feet. Everybody said their feet hurt. Some of those fellows made me sick the way they complained. The next morning (Thursday, April 19th) at 7 AM we again took off and walked until about 10 AM. Then we "dug" in alongside a hill and remained there until about noon. Then the order came down that Co. I was supposed to take off again while the other Companies of the 3rd Battalion stayed back. Our job was to mop up small pockets of resistance which were supposed to have been situated a few miles west of the highway, which the 1st Battalion had already secured. We didn't encounter too much resistance for these German pockets offered very little trouble. They surrendered in "droves". We reached a small town about 6 PM and I'll continue from this point in a later letter.

Sister had asked in one of her letters whether medics receive "combat honors"!!! I explained it in a letter to the folks up home and now I'll explain it to my Lovable Wife. When an infantryman engages the enemy in combat, they receive what is known as the Combat Infantry Badge. This badge they wear above their service ribbons on their left breast. It also gives them a $10 a month bonus. For a long time, they were trying to get some sort of award for the Medic who traveled right with the Infantrymen so in late March they passed a bill (Congress) awarding a "Combat Medical Badge" to all medics attached to an Infantry Regiment in combat. I have already an "order" for this badge. As things stand, we are not receiving the $10 a month bonus but it is before congress now and if that bill passes it will be retroactive since Jan. 1st, 1945. So, we do receive combat honors in every way but not monetary, which is the most important. Ha! Ha! Ha!

Dearest, what do you mean by telling everyone I received that "citation". It doesn't mean that much and people certainly don't care what I receive. I'm sure now that my wife is prouder of that medal than her husband is. Ha! Ha!

So, they think Bill will soon be home!!! What division is he in???? Yes, if he were to come home already, he certainly would be one lucky fellow because he hasn't been overseas long. It looks as though the 10th Mt. Division won't be home for a few months at least so you won't have to "jump out of your pants" yet. Ha! Ha! Darling, you mustn't get so excited in your dreams; you'll have heart failure. Ha! Ha! After thinking that you saw me get off the train and then waking up must give you an awful "let down" feeling, doesn't it???

[Monday] June 18th

If my writing is worse than it usually is, I can offer an excuse. Today while playing softball I was hit on my little finger and it was quite swollen and hurts quite a bit at the moment, but I'll manage to get my letters written. It's just a bruise, by tomorrow it'll be alright. I was the catcher on the winning team. Last night from Grandma I received a box of Billy's Pretzels. Gee those things are delicious.

Here go some more of my experiences. Are you sure you enjoy hearing them?? I left off at 6 PM on Thursday, April 19th. At about this time we hit a small town and sought shelter in some of the buildings until the other companies in the Battalion caught up with us. They arrived around 7:30 PM. On the ridge Northwest of this town, there was still some enemy resistance coming from a group of houses. Well, we were ordered to attack that ridge that very night. This we did and as we were nearing the homes, they opened up on us with machine-gun fire and small arms fire. Well, everybody immediately hit the ground and after engaging in a "firefight" for four hours or more some of our men rushed the houses, threw in hand grenades, and got the Germans but not a single one of our men were hurt. They decided to take things slowly rather than rush right in and have them "mow" us down like flies. In this one house which we took there were Italians living (together with the Germans) and one of the men was injured in the leg. Of course, the first aide man had to fix him up. Well, our whole Battalion dug in on these ridges for the night although it was after 3 AM the next day when I finally laid my head down. Friday morning about 11:00 we were ordered to move to a neighboring ridge and here there were several houses and I was lucky enough to be assigned to one of them. At 4 PM, we again were ordered to move so I never did get to sleep in the house. I think I'll stop here and continue later!!!

So now I'm your Sweetest "Lollypop". Ha! Ha! I guess I just must be a rather sweet person to receive such "sweet" titles!! Now that you drive the car you seem lost the moment you do not have it. I well know how you feel because I can still remember when I had my license taken away for 3 months. Gee, that sort of took a part of my life away because I used my car so much. Gosh, that made me angry when that happened.

Darling, I'm a naughty boy for I should have told you this in yesterday's letter. I have before me the letter you wrote Sat. June 2nd after you returned from Reading and seeing "Without Love" starring Spencer Tracy and Kathryn Hepburn. Well, last Saturday night just as I finished my letters one of the fellows said that an American movie was going to play in the Italian movie house and asked me to go with him. Guess what movie played, none other than "Without Love". Wasn't that a coincidence?? Yes, it was a very good movie. Are you mad at me for going to a movie??

Gee, but that's sad about Norman's wife and her sister. Two sisters received telegrams within a week stating that their husbands had been killed. When you think of that you can see how thankful we can be. Well, we too know how tragic it is to receive such telegrams. Many homes the length and breadth of the country have been saddened by such news but we must always pray and have hope, faith, and courage in the future. There is always a silver lining behind the cloud.

[Tuesday] June 19th

Darling, it is perfectly alright if you wish to discontinue sending me the "standings" because I can follow them in the Stars & Stripes but do not stop sending me the box scores of the Sunday games. The Stars & Stripes never have the box scores in it and I enjoy seeing how the individual men are hitting. Is that okay with my Darling Honey???

We went on this problem today. They took us by truck about 15 miles from here and then we received orders to take a certain number of ridges. Gosh, but it was hot. We even had to dig fox holes when we stopped for a few minutes. We got back rather late. I'm going to bed early tonight because I'm pretty tired.

(second envelope dated June 19th with a copy of "The Stars & Stripes--Mediterranean" with the inscription across the top in ink. ("To Pfc. Luke Snyder-Through the Curtsy of Sweed and Herb")

I'm enclosing a Tuesday Stars & Stripes. In it are the Sports results of Sunday's events. We get the results two days after they take place instead of one day as home newspapers. I'm always trying to get a paper as soon as they come in so that when Tuesday's paper came in a couple of the fellows (Sweed and Herb) got one for me. I had not been here at the time and they laid it on my bunk and had that "inscription" that you'll see on the top. They always kid me about being so anxious about the paper. That fellow Herb Wolfe is from Sunbury, Pa. He knows Frank (Otis's son-in-law) very well. Hope you enjoy the paper.

(Headlines and transcripts from "The Stars & Stripes")

Jap Medium Cities Blasted by B-29s in New Campaign-Four Industrial Centers Hit by 3,000 Tons of Fire Bombs[104]

Triumphal Reception Given Ike in Capitol- "The modest, balding man with the boyish grin came home in triumph today. Traveling with 50 other Yanks in four huge four-motored Skymasters, General of the Army Dwight D. Eisenhower arrived here from Europe this morning to be greeted by a half-million enthusiastic Americans, headed by President Truman".[105]

---

[104] In March the United States Air Force began strategically bombing cities and towns in Japan starting with Tokyo. Over the next five months more than 60 cities were partially destroyed.

[105] A news reel shows General Dwight "Ike" Eisenhower being met by Mamie at the airport and then standing up in a long convoy of jeeps waving to the public masses as he travels down Pennsylvania Avenue.

German Battalion Asks to Fight Japs

15 Poles Plead Guilty to Acts Against Soviets

Trial of Haw-Haw[106] Begins Next Week- "William Joyce, American-born British subject who tried to taunt the British over Nazi radio as Lord Haw-Haw, was formally charged with high treason at ancient Bow Street Court".

Admiral King Urges Peacetime Training- " Commander in Chief of the U.S. Fleet and Chief of Naval Operations Admiral Ernest J. King today joined U.S. Army Chief General George C. Marshall in emphasizing the necessity for compulsory military training in the U.S. during peacetime".

B-29 Hops to Washington From Hawaii in 20 Hours

N.Y. Greets 86th Headed for Pacific- "The 86th (Blackhawk) Division, the first full combat division to return from Europe en-route to the Pacific was welcomed home yesterday in a demonstration unparalleled since World War I".

"With the arrival of 14,289 battle-tested troops, the accelerated redeployment of 3,100,000 veterans of the war against Germany was underway".

"Red, white and blue paint decorated North River piers and service bands blared amid the roar of harbor whistles as three gray transports-James Parker,[107], General Brooke, and General Bliss[108] landed 11,150 officers and men. A fourth

---

Later he speaks to a packed chamber at the Capitol, speaking about the "battles yet to come".

[106] Lord Haw-Haw was the nickname given to the pro-German propaganda broadcaster William Joyce and then later encompassed several other English speaking German broadcasters. Joyce was captured by the British near the end of the war.

[107] Originally the SS Panama built in 1939 it was refitted in 1941 as a troop ship which could hold 2,324 people.

[108] Named after General Raymond Bliss, Assistant Surgeon General of the Army who was instrumental in developing air evacuation in combat.

transport, the Marine Fox, trailed into port several hours later, bringing 173 additional officers and 2,500 enlisted men to Staten island. Four other ships were scheduled to arrive at various metropolitan ports to bring the days total of arriving troops to more than 20,000.

[Wednesday] June 20th

This afternoon our 3rd Battalion Medics had a game with the 2nd Battalion team and as is our custom we lost. The final score was 5-4. I was slated to catch but I didn't want to hurt my finer anymore so I kept score. They had another umpire assigned to the game. My finger is much better but I didn't want to chance reviving the injury.

Here goes a continuation of my doings in Italy. You seem to like what I relate and yet you are "chilled" by what I say. Starting on April 20th, at 4 PM we pushed off and walked for about 30 minutes and then stopped along a side road for about 2 hours. We pushed off again around 7 PM. After walking about 30 minutes artillery started landing in our columns. They were from the Germans Self Propelled guns and gosh they kept landing for about 20 minutes. Co. L suffered the most. A number of their men were killed and wounded. Co. I didn't suffer any casualties again. We were quite lucky. All we got was some smoke from the "shells". Just after this artillery barrage, we came into the Po Valley proper. It was quite dark by now but gosh it was strange to see nothing but flat land after seeing so many hills and mountains. Every field is utilized. One can easily see why the Germans fought so hard for this land; it could easily feed the whole Army. Well, we walked until about midnight after which our company took defensive positions in several fields and "dug in" for the night. That night for the first time we had some German planes overhead. They landed a few bombs and then took off.

The next morning after chow we again took off. We walked and walked and walked and didn't stop until that night at about 8:30 PM. Whew, it seemed we walked right into Berlin. Germans surrendered by the thousands. Our tanks rolled right through and we came along and "mopped" up everything. Gosh, but I was tired that night. I don't believe I ever walked so far in a day. Well, we "dug in" again and that night another German plane was overhead. He again dropped a few bombs and took off. They never came up in the daytime or they'd have been shot down in no time. Well, that was Saturday night, April 21st. At 4 AM Sunday, we again took off. I'll stop here and continue later.

[Thursday] June 21st

No mail from my Sweetheart today. I guess however I can't complain because I was fortunate the last two days to receive sixteen letters from all the folks. This morning about 7:30 my section Sgt. came to me and said that the officers who are having charge of our battalion softball league, which is going to start shortly, want me to be the official scorekeeper for all the games. When the league starts, they will play every day, sometimes afternoons, sometimes evenings. At the end of the week, I will have compiled the team's standings, the batting averages of every player, and the like. Heavens, I hardly ever talked to the Lt. who has it in charge, and yet the Sgt. told me he mentioned me by my first name as the man for the job. This afternoon we had a practice game with Co. K and I saw the Lt. and he insisted I take the job. He'll try and dig up a helper or two so I don't have to be at every game. I kept an official score for this game and gosh, it is amazing how few fellows understand how to score a ball game. When the Lt. saw the score I kept, he insisted that I help him run the league. He called me by my first name and told me to forget he's an officer and call him too by his first name. Now I've deserted both the ranks of umpire and player and now I'm scorekeeper and executive. Ha! Ha! Ha!

Yesterday there were three more soldiers brought into our Medical Section. I heard one of them say he was from Pennsylvania and he told me Tower City. Gosh, that is right near Williamstown where we lived for three years. Darling when I get back, we must all take a trip up through the Lykens Valley and I'll show you where we lived.

[Saturday] June 23rd

Later this morning we were told that college courses at a GI University were going to start soon. Four men from our whole Battalion are all that were allotted for this session. Other sessions will follow and there will be an increase in our allotment for each session. I understand that names will be drawn as to who will be selected. You must have a high school education and IQ of 105 or higher in your Army IQ test.

Here go some more of my experiences in Italy. I left on Sunday morning April 22nd. After receiving our three meals ration, we boarded trucks and took off. We were moving as such a terrific clip that they decided to move our whole Battalion by truck on this day. The tanks were, of course, up ahead of us and were knocking out enemy installations. We took off in trucks and about 10 AM we heard rifle and machine-gun fire up ahead. We were ordered to leave the trucks and seek cover. The head of our Company had run into a German machine-gun nest at a "crossroads". In a few minutes, I heard them yell "Medic" (Company I was leading the convoy), and then I was again dodging machine-gun fire. Ha! Ha! Here I found the wounded man to be none other than our Battalion Commander. He was not wounded badly, just suffering a few scratches and frozen shock. In about 15 minutes the shooting ceased and out came the Germans, some wounded with their hands high. There were also some killed. There were only two of our men wounded and neither was hurt badly. Gosh, but those Germans were scared, they shook all over. Well, we continued and we didn't stop until about 10 PM. During this day we experienced a few such firefights as we had that morning but in each case, the Germans soon came out of their hideouts and gave up. Prisoners literally clogged the roads. They were coming out by the hundreds with their hands up. We didn't even have anyone guarding them. I've never seen so many German prisoners in one day. The thing I'll remember most about this day is the way the Italian people on farms and in the towns came out to greet you. They laughed and threw flowers at you. Others brought out wine, bread, and onions and begged you to take some. They wanted to shake your hand. Others got down and prayed for your presence. Lots cried with joy. We had brought back their freedom and my, oh my, they were happy and glad to see you. All along we would see German equipment and ammunition dumps burning. Fires raged all over the countryside. Our planes were strafing their troops retreat and setting fire to their instillations. Our tanks too were mowing down everything they came across. I realized now that the Germans could not last much longer in Italy. We were just running right through them. Their defense was entirely broken down. I'll continue my story later.

The hospital where the prophylactic station is set up is really a maternity hospital. It is spotlessly clean and it isn't a lot different from ours except that it is lots smaller since it takes care of only maternity cases. Yes, I guess, I'll soon be bringing babies into the world. Ha! Ha!

Yes Darling, aren't you counting your chickens before they're hatched in planning my trip home and how much money I'll need? Ha! Ha! That really would be fine if the Government would pay for our transportation home from camp when we get a furlough. That is almost too much to expect. Ha! Ha!

[Sunday] June 24th

In one of the letters I received from Daddy and Mother yesterday, there was enclosed a few pages from the "Look Magazine" on the correct techniques in playing softball. She said that it might help us medics to win more ball games. Ha! Ha! That game is becoming quite popular. It is by far the most popular sport among soldiers. Volleyball I believe comes second.

Here goes some more of my experiences in Italy. Yes, Sunday, April 22nd we really covered ground. That night we stopped in a field about one or two blocks from the Po River. That night again the Germans had a plane or two overhead but they didn't do any damage to any of the troops. We were told that these planes were piloted by Italian Fascists rather than Germans. He was strafing a lot of troops and would dive real low. Some of our men became terribly frightened and ran for cover. I stayed in my foxhole. After going all day, I was too tired to let a few German planes disturb me. Ha! Ha! The following morning, we again drew our full day's rations and two out of four companies were told to prepare to leave. We boarded trucks and that whole morning we drove through the countryside mopping up small existing German pockets of resistance. At a few times, we were driving right along the Po River. We could see German troop movement on the other side. That is how close we were to the Germans. Here they realized was the only possible defense line they had left, besides the hills of the Alps. After this, we retreated to the place we had "dug in". After eating a couple more cans of C rations we were told that in a few minutes we were going to cross the Po River on small boats that would hold about 12 men each. Just as our first units were starting across, the Germans let go with a concentration of "air-burst" artillery fire. By that, I mean these shells they'd pour over us would explode in the air before they'd hit the surfaces and of course the shrapnel would disperse downward at a terrific speed. A foxhole would be of no help with such fire unless you had a "roof" over it. Well, for about an hour all I heard was "Medic, Medic". Gee, but they inflicted loads of casualties on us for about one hour straight. How some of those air-bursts missed me is nothing short of being a miracle. Finally, we were ordered to withdraw back to our area. About 2:30 PM we retreated about another 2 or 3 blocks and traveled down about a mile or two and then turned back to the river and made another attempt to cross. I'll stop at this point and continue in another letter.

Dearest, there are few yards in Venice. The water is right up against the houses. In fact, some of the steps leading to the doors are underwater. You step right out of the door and into the water. I'm sure that all the houses must have water in them, that is, the cellars at least. I'd think the homes would be very damp all the time.

[Monday] June 25th

Last night at about 7:30 I walked over to the Enlisted Men's Club (no Officers allowed) here in Cividale. It is situated on the third floor of a former school building. They have a writing room, a reading room, and a ping pong table. I was told that practically every night they serve sandwiches or doughnuts and something to drink. Last night they had sandwiches and believe it or not, I had five peanut butter and jelly sandwiches. Ha! Ha! It costs you 50 cents to join. I joined and figured I better get my 50 cents worth the first night because you never can tell when I'd feel like going again. Ha! Ha!

This morning we had an hour and a half lecture on the proper use of certain types of bandages and their application. This afternoon some of the fellows are playing volleyball but I decided to start my daily letters.

Darling, when you say you think I'll be home soon, what do you call soon?? I'm afraid my Darling might be disappointed if she expects me home too soon. I wouldn't be surprised if we remain here or in Austria for two or five months yet.

[Tuesday] June 26th

Gosh, I wonder what has happened to the mail service all of a sudden!!!! Today will be the third consecutive day in which I haven't received any letters. Gosh, but that seems strange. This evening after chow they handed us a questionnaire concerning the Army Educational Program. According to the qualifications I'm qualified to teach some high school and junior college courses so I had to sign up for that. I also said I would like to study at an Army University Study Center. What will happen now, I don't know. Heavens alive, there are so many things coming lately you don't know where you're at. I've signed for the band, to go to college, and to teach high school courses. I'll end up with probably nothing but there is nothing lost anyway. Ha! Ha!

[Wednesday] June 27th

Well, I'm anxious to know whether I'll get any mail today. Last night however I did receive a package from my Dear

Wife. This morning for about 2 hours we had an orientation lecture entitled One World-One War. It had to do with our war against Japan. It was conducted by the Intelligence and Education Section of our Division.

I guess you would like to hear some more of my experiences. I think I stopped when we got ready to cross the Po River for the second time. Well, Co I was the first of our whole Battalion to cross again, as usual. We went over 12 in a boat and while we had quite a bit of artillery fire, none hit in the boat I was in. Just as we all got across, the Germans had caught or rather sighted our place of crossing and started laying on a heavy concentration of fire. Of course, the casualties we received now were on the Northern side of the Po River and we couldn't evacuate them for a few days until we got a bridge built across the river. That was quite rough, too. It is a terrible feeling to be in the middle of a body of water with artillery shells bursting all around you. This day (April 23rd) will also be a day in my life which I'll never forget. After crossing and taking up our positions we were told to dig in. We remained here for about 2 1/2 hours and at 7 PM the order came down to push off again. We walked for about 3 hours and cleared a couple of towns. The Germans were clearing out and retreating rapidly. In one of these towns we cleared, there had been a German hospital situated there. The wounded and sick must have been evacuated that day the way the place looked. Everything was in disorder. At about 10 PM we came upon a few houses. We cleared them and were given them to sleep in for the night. Here we thought we were getting a good place for the night but at 1 AM Tuesday, after about 2 1/2 hours of sleep, they got us up and we pushed off once more. We walked for about three hours and then came upon another small town. Here again, they had us move in with some Italians. At about 5 AM I got to sleep in the attic of a big farmhouse. That same morning at about 9 AM I got up and found out that we weren't scheduled to move out of this place for a couple of days. That noon our Section Sgt. came up to the Company and told me to come back to the Battalion Aid Station for that coming night to rest. He said I could sleep in a barn and there was plenty of straw. The Aid Station was about two miles back from where our Company was. Since our Company was not going to attack that day, he wanted me to come back there to rest for a night. Well, I went to bed rather early on Tuesday night and had a good straw bed for a mattress. I certainly slept quite well that night for the first time in quite a few days. I'll stop here for now and continue later.

Darling in your letter of June 11th you wrote you were cleaning our car and that you were wearing shorts and a halter. Well, honey all I can say is this: you'd better get your "fill" of such clothing because I'm sorry to say that when I get home, I'm afraid you won't be wearing them. Ha! Ha! I still can't say that I like to see you in shorts but as long as I'm not there to see you I'll let you wear them. Ha! Ha! Ha!

Darling, we just had mail call and I received one letter from Mother and that was a back letter. Gosh, but I was so glad to hear from home but I still am anxiously waiting for some mail from my Wife. It is four days now that I haven't received any letters from my Darling. Tomorrow I should certainly get a lot of mail.

[Thursday] June 28th

Gee whiz, but I feel good tonight. Why?? Because I received lots of letters this evening, seven letters in all. This afternoon we medics played Co. L in softball and you guessed it (Ha! Ha!), we lost 15-3. The medics are like Phila. Phillies, only worse! Our manager wants me to get an assistant to keep the official score so I can play myself. He insists that I be their regular catcher. You never knew, did you, that your hubby was a ballplayer? The game was done by 2:40 PM, then we rushed back and changed and went to a U.S.O. show scheduled at 3 PM. It was a pretty good show. Three girls in it danced and sang and three fellows who played some musical instruments. The one fellow who was Master of Ceremonies was, I believe, Roscoe Yates. He played those "Sad Sack" roles in the movies. He also was an exceptional violinist. Is my Honey Darling mad because I saw this U.S.O. performance?? I hope not.

Another page or so on my experiences. I left off on April 24th sleeping in the barn. I got up about 9 AM and quickly managed a couple of airmail letters home. I knew you would be worried about me and I felt much better after mailing them. Doc Nevin censored them right away and mailed them for me. At about noon on Thursday, we pushed off. We walked for about 4-5 hours and at 5 PM trucks came along and we loaded into them. After 2 hours we reached our destination, a field (Ha! Ha!), and were told to dig in for the night. This we did at about 10 PM. Just as I was falling asleep, they got us up and we walked to the nearest town, about a 30-minute walk, and the whole Battalion was put in a building for the night. That was Thursday night, April 26th. I'll stop here for the time being. I'm so glad to hear that your garden vegetables are growing so nicely!!! I only wish that somebody could have worked all of our garden at home. I guess I must put the things out when I get home. You have no idea how ambitious your hubby has become. Ha! Ha! I'll be the busiest man in Berks County.

[Friday] June 29th

Today our whole Battalion has gone on another problem but I was excused from going because of being on C.Q. last night. I'm taking care of the building seeing to it that everything is in order. As a result, I do not have much to do today.

As you have probably seen in the paper nine Divisions from the European Theater of Operations have been assigned to go to the Pacific while others have been assigned to the occupation Armies. Nothing is definite about the Divisions in Italy. I think the 34th will soon be assigned to the Pacific; the 85th and the 88th will go home and be redeployed while the 91st and 10th have not been given a definite assignment. General McNarney stated that by Jan 1st there would be only 2,500 GIs in Italy. One division he said, would be assigned to the Trieste Area. At the moment the 91st and 10th are in this area. Who will get the permanent assignment is the big secret. Ha! Ha!

I bet you all "razzed" Aunt Marion about giving Grandpa cascara instead of cough medicine. Ha! Ha! That cascara is really quite a laxative. We use that same stuff in the Army for constipation.

[Monday] July 2nd

Honey Bunch, things certainly do happen fast. I bet you can't possibly imagine where I am or what I'm doing. Ha! Ha! Gee whiz, it's a long story but I'll tell you where I am. I'm in Florence, Italy and I'm going to attend Army University Center here. I'll bet you hardly can believe it. Well, neither could I when they first told me. I'm terribly sorry but I was unable to write either Sat. or Sun. The whole time was spent on coming here and getting my room and the like. Well, I'll start at the very beginning and tell you the whole story, okay??

On Saturday we had several games of volleyball. At about 10:15 we were going to get paid for June. Sometime this month our Medical Section was planning to have a party of some sort and on payday, we were asked to contribute a dollar or more for the purchase of food and drinks for this party. Well, our Section Sgt. asked me to collect from the fellows as they got paid. While I was doing this, he came running up to me and said "Say, Luke, if you were able to go to the University what courses would you like to take?" He seemed to be very much in a hurry so I told him quickly. After I had collected from everybody, I saw him and he told me that I was one of those selected to go but he had no idea when I'd go. At 11 AM our Medical Section was going to have a softball game among ourselves. When I returned to our building, at noon, I was told that the order came down that I was supposed to be ready to leave at 2 PM. Gee whiz, that really caught me unexpectedly. I was going to leave and go to Florence to a University and I had no idea what to take with me and what to leave behind. Well, everything I thought I'd need and want I put in my barracks bag. I found out that another medic and a fellow from Co. K were the three men to go from our whole Battalion. This other Medic also had four years of college, a nice fellow from Chicago. The fellow from Co. K has had one year of college at the University of California. The orders read that I am on Temporary Duty for four weeks starting Sunday, July 1st. The truck came about 4 PM to take us and just before we left the mail came in and was given to me. One thing I don't like is that I won't be receiving any mail for the next few days. Any mail I get now will be forwarded from my outfit so will take a few days longer to get to me.

We got to Bologna around 11 PM Sat. after driving a long time. We had a flat tire on the way and with these tires, they have on the Army trucks, it is a job to change a tire. After sweating and getting ourselves all dirty we managed to get it changed. When we got to Bologna we went to the Officer in charge of "billeting" for soldiers in "transient". We got rooms in an apartment house that was really clean and had beds with "white sheets". Gosh was that something!! We didn't pay a single thing for the rooms. We were up around 9:15 and then on our way to Florence. Gosh, but the roads were terribly mountainous, full of curves and the roadbed itself was full of ruts. I thought my insides would turn upside down. Ha! Ha! Ha! We arrived in Florence at about 3:30 PM and went to the rest camp I was in before and had a good hot shower. We then went to the University,[109] was issued our bedding, cots, and were placed in a room. The fellow from K Company and I shared a room. Around 5 PM we had a formation and the President of the University talked to us. He's Brigadier General Tate. He told us that high scholastic standards must be maintained or you'll "flunk" and be returned to your outfit. I'm staying in Room 103 in "Citadel" Hall. Classes will not start until July 9th so we'll probably be here for about 5 weeks. The Red Cross has a nice lounge and writing room here and that is where I'm writing this letter. This University was built in 1937, under Mussolini of course, and was an Aeronautics School. When we took over it was turned into the 24th General Hospital. It is a very fine place and I consider myself very lucky to have been able to come. If they offer "postgraduate" courses I'll work for my "Masters" degree in Chemistry. If they don't, I'm going to take up

---

[109] The Army University Center was set up to help transition soldiers from Army life to University attendance and students generally attended for one term. It was also a starting point for racial integration in the military.

Political Science History and Social Studies. If they have a band or orchestra, I'll join that too. The University is on the outskirts of town in one of the many parks in Florence. I might add that in case our outfit leaves Italy before the month is up, I'll be called back but if it just moves within the country itself, I'll stay right here.

[Tuesday] July 3rd

I hope that tomorrow we'd all have a day off because of Independence Day. I see by the posters around the campus that there will be quite a celebration in Florence. The barbershop and the University post office are in the same building we are staying in. Say, my Sweetheart, in one of the letters you mentioned that Sister was going to give you some oil to put on your skin so that you won't burn red!! Did you use that stuff when you were "getting your suntan"? I am so amused at my Darling trying to get a suntan!! Ha! Ha!

No, My Sweetheart, as yet I have not written to Ed's parents or his girlfriend. I must have mislaid his parent's address but I still have his girlfriend's address. I guess one really should write but it is so difficult to

write such a letter. I thought maybe when I'd get home you and I could drive out to his folk's place one day and see them personally. He told me his parents would so much like to have him bring me to his home because Ed was always mentioning me. I'm sure, neither he nor I had a better friend in the Army than each other.

Yes, we will definitely visit the Yankee Stadium in the near future. I've always wanted to see that immense structure and there is no use waiting any longer. I see that the Phillies won a doubleheader on Sunday from Cincinnati!! What in the world has happened to them?? Ha! Ha! I also saw that Fitzsimmons has resigned and that Herb Pennock has signed

Ben Chapman, one of their pitchers, as the manager for the rest of the year. Poor Phillies!!!

There are many, many German prisoners working around the University. In fact, they do just about everything. They clean and scrub your building's floors plus lawn cleaning and fixing up. They are the permanent K.P.s in the kitchen. Outside of the head cook all the other cooks and all the K.P.s are German War prisoners and believe it or not the food is very good. On Sunday evening I ate my first meal here and when the first fellow put the meat on my try it was such a small piece, so I told him I wanted some more. He readily gave it to me. All the helpings they gave you are so small. Of course, they give you as much as you want if you ask them but they seem so surprised at how much we Americans are given to eat. I remarked to the fellow next to me that I guess they were used to handing out such small portions in their own Army. Ha! Ha! Last night they had ice tea for a beverage and when I told him it was good, in German, he was so happy and said he made it. By this morning all the PWs must have known I spoke German because they all bid me the time of day and gave me exceptionally huge potions. I'm stuffed from all I ate this noon. We had spaghetti and meatballs, and gosh it was very good, and to think I hated spaghetti before I came in the Army. Ha! Ha!

Honestly, I can still hardly make myself believe that I'm here in Florence and going to school. It happened so quickly that it takes a while for it to "soak in". Gee whiz, all the fellows here seem terribly smart. They might have pretty tough courses from what I hear. I guess I'll have to learn to study all over again.

[Wednesday] July 4th

This morning it was announced that all University activities would cease for the day and that all students could have passes to go in town until midnight tonight. This afternoon I went into town with another Medic by the name of Carl. There was supposed to be a U.S.O. show at 2:30 at one of the theaters in Florence starring Jinx Falkenburg,[110] the movie actress but at 1:30 when we got there, they were already standing in line so we didn't stay. The same actress was supposed to play an exhibition tennis match on the main tennis court at 4 PM, but it was so hot we decided not to go. As a result, I passed up an opportunity to see a movie actress. Ha! Ha! This fellow Carl was anxious to buy a pair of swimming trunks and after he bought them, we decided to come back here. According to the program, there is going to be another U.S.O. in town tonight, together with movies, a street dance and band concert plus fireworks from 11:30 to midnight. Most of the fellows have gone in town but I'd much rather stay here and write my darling letters. So, as you see my "Fourth" has been very uneventful.

Why would I think my Darling is naughty simply because she does a little complaining once in a while?? You know they often say that a person wouldn't be human if he wouldn't complain once in a while. Ha! Ha! Are you still having such hot weather?? By this time, I guess, you'll be more used to it!!

I'll bet Sister feels relaxed since her exam is over. She's a great one. She always says she'll flunk and she turns up with an "A" anyway. She puts a lot of work into her courses. Yes, Ruth, you must convince Sister that she should treat Dick

---

[110] Eugenia (Jinx) Falkenburg was a model/actress born in Barcelona, Spain. In 1940 she was picked to be the first "Miss Rheingold" for Rheingold Beer. She traveled extensively on the USO tours entertaining troops.

271

much better. Gosh, he's a swell fellow and he always enjoyed coming up to our house.

Dearest, I don't want to find a scale anywhere for fear by stepping on it I might receive some "bad" news. Ha! Ha! I really think I'll have to cut out one meal and eat but twice a day. I should be able to tell you what courses I'll be taking soon. I think the men from "Citadel" matriculate tomorrow.

[Thursday] July 5th

Well, today I matriculated. Gosh, till I had inquired into everything and finally selected the courses I'm going to take and the like, it consumed my whole day. Well, for this first session they are not offering any postgraduate courses in Physical Science but they felt that maybe by the next session they would and if so, they'd be very glad to have me work with them. You are required to take three courses. I'll have a class course each weekday. Plus an hour of physical education is required each day. Here is the schedule of the courses I'm taking.

1) 8-8:50 American Government 2) 9-9:50 Principle Sociology 3) 10-10:50 Physical Education 4) 11-11:50 free Hour 5) 1-1:50 Economic Geography. The rest of my day, except from 5-5:30 when we have close order drill, I have to myself. This first session ends August 4th, so I'll be here at least that long.

[Friday] July 6th

My Dearest Heart Throb,

How do you like that salutation?? Gee but I hope she is not mad at me now!!! Honestly, you have no idea how anxious I am to receive my mail. Right before I started your letter, I inquired at the post office for another change of address card and filled it out and mailed it so in case the first one got lost there will be another one on its way. I'm keeping my fingers crossed, hoping that by tomorrow I'll receive some mail.

My Darling, do you remember what happened 52 weeks ago today??? Last year at this time we were having such a good time in New York City. But on Friday when we came home, we had that "little" trouble with that patrolman. You know I can still see us stopping at that refreshment stand and having some Root Beer and Hot Dogs and then we decided that you should take the wheel for a while and, lo and behold, didn't we run into the "cop". Did you really think he'd "take us in"?? I guess we are pretty good actors, aren't we?? Ha! Ha! I must admit I didn't feel too good there for a while, how about you??? Well, it turned out okay. And now my Sweetheart is a licensed driver and a very good one at that.

My Sweetheart, it does seem very peculiar that the government has sent your parents Howard's back pay plus his insurance money for the months from Feb. to Dec. The back pay amounted to over $500 in all, didn't it??? I had been wondering if they were getting any insurance money. Does the government send a certain amount each month until the value of the policy has been reached? The only explanation I can see for paying both his pay and the insurance is that when a soldier is listed missing his pay continues and since according to the War Department, they had made an error in the first telegram, they feel as if the back pay should be paid.

I probably will receive the Bronze Star while I'm here at the University. That is, they will receive it for me. I understand that a parade was soon going to be held and I was probably to be given my "Star". However, in my absence from my unit, it will probably be given to our "Doc" and I'll get it from him. I'm glad if that takes place rather than having to stand before a whole Battalion or Regiment and have some high-ranking officer pin it on you. I'm much too modest for that sort of thing. Ha! Ha!

Well today, tomorrow, and Sunday we are having a few days of leisure until the work will begin. The order came down that we must put a minimum of three hours of work on our courses every night. They'll be quite lucky if I'm putting that much time into my studies. Ha! Ha! Of course, it depends on how much they are going to cover and how difficult they will make each course but I'll be darn if my letters home are going to suffer because of school work. Ha! Ha!

[Saturday] July 7th

Today is exactly one week since I've received any mail so you can imagine how I feel. But I know you all have been writing every day so I'll get quite a stack of letters and believe me I'll feel 100% better. Yesterday after completing my letter writing who should be walking over to me but a fellow that I had basic with at Camp Barkeley. He said he left for Italy on Jan 13th and docked at Naples on the 23rd. He's a pharmacist and he has quite the job at some "rear echelon" hospital, but here's the catch. When he was selected to come up here, his Commanding Officer told him that he could expect to be recalled in a week or two because his outfit is going directly to the Pacific. Isn't it strange how you can leave a fellow at one place and then meet again over 4000 miles from there about 8 months later?

This morning I picked up my textbooks; you know the government is spending quite a bit of money on this educational program. Late this morning we were given a PX ration card. We have a regular PX on-campus only things are rationed and you can only buy so much of a certain thing. They punch your ticket when you buy things. You can only buy one pack of cigarettes in a day, 1 can of beer in a day, and one pack of gum every day. The PX just got in a lot of supplies and the line of soldiers waiting to purchase things is about a half-mile long. By golly, I can't in the world see what could be important enough to stand in line for that long. Ha! Ha!

Darling, I'm convinced that everything does happen to you. Believe me, I laughed and laughed and laughed some more when I read your experience concerning the trouble you had with the car horn. That car of yours is giving you loads of trouble lately. I can remember that same thing happened to me only once before in all my driving. But please don't let anything like that upset or worry you. It just adds more excitement and diversion to one's life, how about it???? Ha! Ha! Ha! How is the radiator working?? Does she still get hot for you??? Does the motor sound better to you than it did when you thought it sounded "louder" after you had it "fixed"? I'm sure it's cleaner since you take care of it more than when I was home.

The more I think of things I've been through in the last six months the more thankful I am. When you were right up there in the thick of it a fellow didn't really have time to think of the danger he was in. He just kept his wits about him and carried on but now when one can recall all the things that happened it seems like a miracle that you came out of it in one piece.

Darling, your hubby has a bone to pick with his wife. Now don't worry, he isn't angry but he thinks she should have voted at the Primary Election on the 19th of June. Since my wife can drive the car, she has no excuse to offer even if her father didn't feel like voting. I guess I'm a great fellow in that respect, but it's our duty to vote. It is part of our great democracy and we must show a continued interest in it. This war should show us more so than anything else that we must do all we can to keep our democracy alive. We must fight for that always and we all should cast our ballot every election day. I say that to everyone, no matter how he or she votes. Now you'll make your hubby very happy if you be sure to vote in the future.

[Sunday] July 8th

Well, still no mail. If they only knew how anxious I am to receive mail, they wouldn't be so slow in sending it to me. I keep "hounding" the mail clerk so much that he'll bring it to my room as soon as any mail comes. Ha! Ha!

Well, as you probably guessed, your hubby was at church services this morning. We had a guest chaplain. He was a Lt. Colonel and is head chaplain of this particular training command. The regular chaplain, Capt. Daniel was also there. Tonight at 8 PM there will be a service for the German Prisoners of War and all those who understand German are invited as it would show good fellowship. They also will hold devotional services every Monday thru Friday for 15 minutes at 7:30, right after chow, and before classes start.

Here, in one room of the Red Cross lounge, they sew and make alterations to your clothing. I brought in my O.D. shirt and will have them sew on my Divisional Insignia. I never bothered having it sewn on because I frequently got different clothes at the shower unit. We only had one set from the time we came over until the end of May. It's definite now that we will not be issued "suntans". [111] They claim there is a shortage of "suntans" and that is why all units are not wearing them.

Last evening the fellows I came down with went to the PX to get their rations so I went along. I bought the beer and

---

[111]These were soldier uniforms that were made of lighter weight tan fabric worn during the summer months.

cigarettes that were allotted to me and then sold them back to these other fellows. I bought some Mennen Talcum powder, some foot powder, and a can of fruit juice. This noon while I was eating, a fellow from the 10th Mt. Division came up and said, did you hear the latest rumor on where we're going? He said we're being pulled back to Montecatini, which was the city we were in for a few days of rest back in March. I don't think there is any truth in it, I'm positive we'll be here until fall.

I saw on the bulletin board that on August 2nd and 3rd we will have our final examinations. By the "Stars and Stripes" this morning I see the 85th Division is going home very soon. When that division hits the states, they are going to deactivate it. They have transferred all "high point" men from other divisions into it and also transferred low point fellows into outfits that are not going home right away. Gosh but our Air Forces are really hitting Japan hard!! 600 planes plus fighters took part in one of the last raids.

[Monday] July 9th

Gee Whiz, Darling, but they have piled the work on us at the Study Center. All three of my instructors have warned their classes that we'll have frequent examinations. Since there will be only 20 hours of lecture in this first session, they are going to cover ground. In Economic Geography we are going to meet two more hours a week besides our regular hours.

Well, still no mail!!!! I can't understand where all my mail is. I've gone to everyone who might have something to do with the mail situation but all they tell me is that it just hasn't come in yet. Nine days have gone by without mail.

This afternoon at 3:00 the University Study Center was finally dedicated by the Commanding General of the 5th

Army, Lt. General Lucian Truscott. Major General Hays, the commanding General of the 10th Mt. Division, was also at the ceremony. Also attending was a band from a nearby Replacement Depot, who rendered the military selections.

[Tuesday] July 10th

Gee, but you have no idea how good your husband feels this evening. I received some mail. My hopes and prayers were answered. Here's the funny thing. There are mailboxes on the 2nd floor of our hall; that is a mailbox for every letter of the alphabet. I went up to the mailboxes immediately after classes were over and gosh, I had no mail. I felt so disappointed. When I came into my room, there I found my mail on my bed. Here Carl Larson (the other Medic) had gotten mine when he went up for his earlier. Gee but I threw down my books and tore into it. Ha! Ha! I received a total of nine letters. I'm just "bubbling over" with joy tonight because I received some mail from my Darling.

I have two tests scheduled for Friday of this week. So far, I like American Government the best of all. Honestly that stuff really "comes" to me. I can "raddle" off answers to these questions before he can get them out of his mouth. Ha! Ha! Dearest, how would you like a politician or rather a husband in public life???? I wouldn't be surprised if I might seek some public office. I like government and everything connected with it. After all, we "veterans" are going to have a lot of say in national life after the war. Now don't become alarmed, Honey Darling. Your husband is just dreaming, I guess. Ha! Ha! Ha!

That is perfectly O.K., my Darling, for not telling me the results of the Primary Election. Daddy and Mother gave me the results. That was of great interest to me. Our man was nominated for Judge, but not for Prothonotary. Now my

Dearest will make me very happy if she goes to the polls in November. I want my wife to take an interest in those things. How about it??

About that argument you say you, Sister and Mother had; my Honey Bunch was entirely right. I certainly did have to pay for all those PX rations. I'm afraid the government would go broke if they gave every soldier $3.20 worth of food and the like every two or three weeks. I can't see where Mother and Sister got that idea. When an outfit is in combat or on the front lines, he gets a bar of candy (a penny bar) and a pk. of cigarettes every day for no cents, plus a bar of soap, toothpaste, and the like every once in a while. But now that the conflict is over, we pay for all our things but get much more of it.

I haven't been relating any of my experiences in the last week's letters. I've been filling my letters with my experiences which are taking place at the moment. It feels very strange to be going to "college" again but I couldn't think of a better way of spending my time while waiting for shipment.

So, Whitey Kurowski has another "son". Yes, he seems to be going quite well again this year with the St. Louis Cardinals. I see they are only 1 1/2 games out of first but the Browns are quite disappointing to me.

[Wednesday] July 11th

Well, I got some bad news today. I'll have a term paper to prepare in that American Government course; probably two. This first one must be in by July 20th. The topic I'm writing on is a mighty good one though: "The Nomination and Election of our President". I can write a 1000-word paper on that without even consulting a reference. Ha! Ha! The only thing I don't like is the fact that it takes time. Next Monday we must also hand in a paper in this course Economic Geography. My subject there is "Forest Conservation". What a life!!! It seems this Army is just not satisfied unless they keep you busy.

I'm glad to hear you received our bond for April. By golly, they are two months behind. Do you have an idea how much money we have in bonds??? Of course, I'm figuring at their maturity value when I estimated about $1200. I think we have about that much since you bought a $100 bond with that income tax refund of 1943, didn't you?

Dearest, the Austrian border, I believe, is only about 60 or 80 miles from Cividale. In fact, it might not even be that far. Darling, why don't you want to take the car to work on Friday and Saturday??? Are you afraid of having more dents put in your fenders?? Ha! Ha! If it's more convenient for you to use the car you be sure to use the car. Gee, your hubby is laying down the "law" isn't he?? I guess you think I'm being pretty strict. Darling, you know I'm just kidding, you do exactly as you please!!

I'm surprised that you would like it if something was the matter with me. So, you don't want me in good physical condition?? Ha! Ha! Well, I'm afraid I can't do anything about it. Every time they have ever examined me, I'm in 100% shape. Must I laugh; you know I was supposed to have a touch of tuberculosis, an overactive heart, and flat feet, and even despite all that they put me in the 10th Mt. Division, probably the most "rugged" division in existence and what is even more amazing I've taken all they threw at me and I'm still hale and hardy. Ha! Ha! Ha!

If I remember correctly Sister told me in her letter that James said he read that the 10th Division received the Presidential Citation. Well, I've been told something about that from a Divisional Officer who is here attending the

University. Two Battalions out of the total of nine in the whole Division were originally accepted for the Presidential Citation and it was going to be formally announced but at the last moment, Major General Hays held up the citation and is now trying to get the whole Division a citation. This is mighty hard to do. This Officer then said that the two Battalions which had already been accepted for the Citation were the 3rd Battalion of the 87th Regiment and the 3rd Battalion of the 85th Regiment. So now I know that officially we are regarded as one of the top Battalions. I'm sure no Battalion could have had as rough going as we had on the 14th and 15th of April. Our Battalion according to this officer had more men killed and wounded than any other outfit. I guess we just must have hit the most "stoutly" defended terrain. The 85th Regiment had more men killed and missing in action than the other two Regiments.

Darling, you mustn't get mad at what I wrote about the Germans firing upon us. So, you actually saw "red". Ha! Ha! Here's the comical part of it. Cases have been known where Americans have also fired on German Medics. In fact, one of our infantrymen killed a German Medic. We ordered him to raise his hands and move behind our lines but the "bum" ran off so we let him have it. Of course, we are allowed to shoot to kill when an attempt to escape is made, even if they're Medics.

[Thursday] July 12th

I'm writing immediately after evening chow and I hope you'll forgive me for writing only a short letter but tomorrow I have two examinations plus a lot of work to do in my third course, so I'll spend my whole evening studying. I'm just about the happiest man in the world this evening because I received the mail this afternoon. I got fourteen letters, seven from my Dearest and Most Wonderful Wife, plus seven from the folks up home.

[Friday] July 13th

I hope you haven't experienced any ill luck this far because today is Friday the 13th. Three months ago, we also had a Friday the 13th, April 13th. I'll never forget those days! Today is another swelter and I mean that too. A fellow just had to sit down and he is perspiring. The announcement was posted on the bulletin board that any student desiring to stay here for another four-week session should apply before 6 PM today. In the application, they wanted to know how many points you have. I don't know why they wanted to know that!! I figure I might as well be learning something while I'm here, don't you??

I'm disgusted. Last night I prepared for two tests today and I didn't have a single one. The one "prof" postponed it until Monday because he wanted to cover some more material. The other "prof" decided he'd rather have us write a paper to be handed in on Monday. I'll have my hands full for Monday!! This morning I played volleyball, next week I might play something else. I understand they have 50-75 horses here and that you can go horseback riding. It's something new for me but I like horses a lot and would like to learn how. Then when I get home, we'll both go riding. If I could find someone to keep our horses, we'd buy a few. I'm a great fellow. I'm talking about doing so many things, am I not???

Both Harold and Bill you say are in the 86th Division!! Yes, they are certainly getting nice furloughs. I guess we could enjoy a 30 to 45-day furlough, couldn't we?? Gosh, that's too good to even think about.

[Saturday] July 14th

This noon I received eleven letters and one of them was from Francis. Gee, but I was glad to hear from Francis. According to his address, he is still in the same outfit he had always been in. He mentioned that he was stationed 31 miles from Brussels, Belgium.

This morning we had a good lecture on an "orientation" subject. The man teaching it happened to mention that he was from the Eastern part of Pennsylvania. After the hour was up, I asked him where he was from and he said he's from Reading, Pa. He and his wife have a summer home in that back road from Shoemakersville, just a short distance above Kindt's Corner. He taught school at Hershey and lives on W. Greenwich St. in Reading. He said he knew my Father but he probably wouldn't remember him. He's going to come to my room sometime and have a long talk. He is, I'd say, at least 36 years old, graduated from F&M in 1930, and has been overseas for 34 months, but he had a furlough over Christmas. He has some office job in the "rear" area somewhere. In the excitement, being in a hurry to leave, I forgot to ask his name.

You know, I can teach or rather supervise the Organic Chemistry laboratory work here at the University next month if I want to and if I remain here. They are in need of "profs" in physical science and he said I'd just be the fellow they are looking for. Gosh, a fellow is offered so many things; he doesn't know what to do. Ha! Ha!

My Darling, I've heard very reliable rumors that the 10th Division was going to move south. If this is true, I don't know what it possibly could mean.

Guess what, I went horse-back riding!! My roommate came into the room this morning and said, "Say, Luke, I've signed you up for a horse this afternoon at 3 PM. I want

somebody to go riding with me and I'm sure you'll go along."
I said, 'Just a moment, I can't ride a horse." But he insisted I
go with him and when I got there, I asked the fellow in charge
of the stable for a real "gentle" horse. He said they all were
pretty full of life. Holy smokes, I said to this fellow, I'm
going back to my room, I can't ride an animal. By this time
about eight more fellows had come and were getting their
horses, a whole group signs up for certain hours and they all
go out together. Well, I struggled on my horse and as soon as
I got on top he wanted to "run" off but I pulled on the reins
and he stopped. Ha! Ha! All the horses were walking nicely
along and there was nothing to it but when we got away from
the university and out in the open the rest of the group started
at a fast "gallop" and my horse wanted to go too. Well, I gave
him the "reins" and he really took off. Gosh, I thought surely
I'd fall off. Finally, I got on to the whole thing and I caught up
with the group. These fellows had all "ridden" many times
before and here I was just a rookie, but gosh I soon learned
how to control my horse. We trotted a while and then
someone got the idea we should have a little race. I surely
wasn't going to get in a race but they insisted I get in it. Well,
I figured I could stay on so if the horse wanted to run, I'd let
him. We came upon a nice dirt road that looked fairly level
and they took off. My horse didn't start so well but finally
started to gain. Gee whiz, I thought I'd fall off that horse's
back but I braced my knees and let the horse go. Finally, I
passed two other horses; the dust was so thick I hardly could
see where I was going. Finally, I kicked the horse a little with
my heels and then we passed the other horses and we stayed
out in front until we all stopped. I rode a horse and even raced
him was certainly a great surprise to me. It is certainly funny
what a person can do if he makes up his mind on that thing. I

have no ill effects either except that my "rear" seems a little sore. Ha! Ha! I think I'll refrain from that sport for a while.

Sister tells me that Bill had to cry because of the thought of going to the Pacific. I guess that is not a pleasant thought to think of but if I'd be home, I'd be too happy to cry no matter if I knew I was going to the Pacific. I think of those guys who go to the Pacific and don't get home.

P.S. Darling, I've received your letter about not having to wear stockings to work if your legs are suntanned. I don't know what to say about that. Your hubby certainly will not scold his wife for not wearing stockings but I guess he is still somewhat of an "old fogey" for if I were to see my wife go away without stockings, I'm sure I would not like it. But now here's what you do. Since it is so hot at home I can't mind if you fail to wear stockings once in a while but don't get into the bad habit of doing without them all the time because your hubby still likes a woman who maintains her womanliness and I think that bare legs do not become a woman. Now please don't let me discourage you, my Dear, you just go bare-legged when it is so hot but always remember that you still look more the wonderful woman you are when you have stockings on. How about it??? Please do not think too ill of your husband, after all, it is only his opinion.

Love & Kisses Luke XXXXX's

[Sunday] July 15th

This morning I attended church services and the chapel was overflowing with soldiers. The chaplain announced that next week it would be held in a larger auditorium. This afternoon I wrote my paper on Sociology and studied for my examinations. Has the 10th Mt. Division hit the headlines or made the news broadcasts on the radio the last day or two??

[Monday] July 16th

My Sweetheart, I didn't know whether I should tell you this or not but I decided to. The way things look now the 10th Mt. Division will come back to the States before too many months pass. Things have suddenly taken a change. Our Division was supposed to remain in the Trieste Area as an occupation outfit but that job has been assigned to the 34th Division. In my letter of a few days ago I mentioned the fact that the rumors had it that the 10th was going to move "south". Well, they have moved south and guess where they've moved-right here in Florence, only about 300 yds. from the University. It is supposedly a redeployment area. I've heard that the fellows from the Division that are attending the University will soon be called back to their outfits. Gosh, don't things happen quickly. Here I was looking forward to spending a few weeks here and now I'll probably be leaving in a day or two. Ha! Ha! Ha! I said this in yesterday's letter and I'll say it again in this one, don't send any more packages. Tonight sometime, I might walk down to where our Battalion is located and see what the situation is. I guess you might see me much before you had anticipated. Do you mind??? The thought of getting home really thrills me but I won't believe I'm "home" until I hit the good old U.S.A. Ha! Ha! Ha!

You tell me Walt is coming home!!! Gee, he's been overseas for some time, hasn't he?? I believe his two brothers are both out of the country too. You mentioned in your letter of June 24th that 45 Divisions were mentioned in the New York Times and what they were going to do but nothing mentioned of the 10th. I'd be willing to bet that in the papers of July 15th the 10th Mt. Division was mentioned. How nearly right was I???

Believe me, you have a very good idea there my Honey Bunch about going picnicking when I come home. I guess you can't get batteries for our radio, now can you?? I'll have to have a radio with me so that I can hear the baseball games. My dear still knows how much her hubby likes baseball games.

[Tuesday] July 17th

Yesterday I received my mail around 5:30 PM and I received in one of your letters all those wonderful pictures. Gosh, but was I glad to see them. I carry them with me all the time and even during my class period I'm constantly getting them out and admiring them. Gosh, but that it is such a very good picture of my Honey in her blue dress, and Darling you won't have to worry about me getting a divorce because of that picture where you "display" your legs. Ha! Ha! I was so glad for all the pictures of the folks too and of Flush. I'm so glad you managed to get a picture of Daddy. I never had a single picture of him.

My Sweetheart, you have been pestering me so much lately for the thing that happened on April 15th. All the "gory" details I'd rather relate personally but my unit received my Bronze Star Ribbon and the Citation. They sent me a "summary" of this citation and I'll pick them up when I return to my outfit. Here is what the statement says that they sent me:

"Luke M. Snyder 33837555, Private First Class Medical Department 85th Mt. Infantry, United States Army: For heroic achievement in action on the 15th of April 1945 near Castel d' Arno, Italy. In the attack on a strongly defended mountain objective, Private First Class Snyder performed his duties as a Company Aid Man with high courage, determination, and concern for the welfare of his comrades saving many lives and preventing much suffering and pain. At one time while continuously treating wounded men he heard the cry for help, and at the height of deadly mortar barrage immediately set out to reach a wounded man, treat him, and evacuate him to a covered position. His tireless efforts and unflinching devotion to duty were essential factors in the full success of his organization's work. Private First Class Snyder justly merits high praise and respect for such an inspiring performance of a humane mission. He entered the military service from Allentown, Pennsylvania."

By Command of Major General Hays

They surely did overemphasize my work when they wrote out that Citation, didn't they?? The thing that happened at the "height of that deadly mortar barrage" is what I'll never forget. It always makes me feel as though I'm the luckiest individual in the world. I'm certainly thankful for getting out of it all fine. That statement should be enough of an explanation, anything else you want to know I'll explain when I return home.

The fellow who teaches American Government has already corrected our exams and he gave me a grade of 98%. There are no marks on the paper so I don't know why he didn't give me 100%. Ha! Ha! He remarked that 98% was the highest grade and that as a rule he was rather displeased with the papers because there were too many "flunks" and I thought the test was easy.

Naturally, I don't mind, in the least, if you visit V. Bowman. I can well imagine how glad she would be to have company especially at such a time as she is now experiencing.

[Wednesday] July 18th

I guess you are wondering why I'm writing at 1:30 PM. Well, things are starting to happen. Tomorrow morning all the men of the 10th Mt. Division who are attending the

University are going to leave and return to their outfits. The "special" notice was posted on the bulletin board about 11:30 this morning, so it looks as though we are definitely leaving the country and undoubtedly headed for the good old U.S.A. It seems as though the papers and the radio make announcements to that effect whenever a Division is headed for the States and when they arrive. The announcement stated that we were supposed to get a "clearance" slip from the Adjutant Generals Office and then turn in all our equipment (books etc.) that we got since we were here. Now listen to this Darling, this may be the last letter I'm able to write for some time. I'm sure for the next few weeks before we leave there will be much for us to do. If I were you, I would refrain from writing when you receive this letter because I'll probably be on my "way". The thought of seeing "home" again just thrills me. Oh, happy day!!!!

Say, was R. Moser home over the 4th of July??? You mentioned that he was expected home. I presume he is in the hospital, Mother said in Atlantic City. I'm wondering just how badly he was hurt? Let's hope he wasn't hurt too badly!!!

What do you think of those Chicago Cubs?? They are the surprise of the National League. Of course, I still think the Cards will win out but it will be pretty close this year. Your New York Giants are definitely out of the running. Ha! Ha! My Brownies are way down in 6th place and yet are 6 1/2 games out of first place.

[Friday] July 20th

This letter will be the last one I'll be able to write until I see you in person. The order came down that tomorrow morning all mail would have to be done. We moved to our outfit yesterday and a lot of the things which the outfit had done in the last three, four days I had to do yesterday and "catch up" so to speak. The latest rumors say we're going to leave sometime on Sunday and head for "Naples" by train. We'll probably ride in cattle cars. We'll get on the boat there. Things are really on a terrific clip.

I turned in lots of my clothing and equipment and guess what, they gave us one pair of "suntans" but we are not allowed to wear them until we get off the boat in the U.S.A. I was left under the impression that when we hit the states, we'll receive two more sets of "suntans". I hope so because these O.D.s are too hot to wear in summer. This morning we had a physical examination. It was the most thorough exam I've had since I'm overseas. I hear that if you did not come up to a certain standard you would not go home with your outfit. Two of our medics failed and they are staying over here. They're not too well pleased but in the long run, they will be just as well off. This afternoon we turned in all our Allied Military Currency except what we might want to spend before boarding the boat. We'll get U.S. Currency while crossing the Atlantic. Yes, my Sweetheart, it looks as though you'll see your hubby before too many weeks pass by.

Dearest did you really feel that sick when you saw in the paper that I'd be here until November?? Gee, but you poor dear!!! It seems that no matter where I'll be you won't feel right but I want my Darling to forget all about the distant future and think only of the wonderful time we are going to have when I come home. Is that a promise??? Now that's an order from your boss!!!

Sister sent me that newspaper clipping about my "Bronze Star". Who in the world put that in the paper?? I don't like to see my name in the headlines. Ha! Ha! Speaking of that, yesterday when I came back to my unit, they gave me my Bronze Star and my Ribbon. Gee but the medal is nice. The Regimental Co. Officer had wanted to pin it on me back in

Cividale but since I was here at the University, he gave it to our Section Sgt. instead. Yes, whoever wrote that article for the Reading Times really "slings the bull". Ha! Ha!

Darling, I'm so glad you had a pleasant 4th of July and found someone to go swimming with you at the Kutztown swimming pool. Gee, but my Darling must have a suntan by this time!! Well, what is so wonderful about having a suntan?? I can't see that your skin looks any nicer if it's brown, red, or white. Ha! Ha! My Wife's beautiful no matter what color she is. Boy, am I hungry for some delicious Hot Dogs!! I'm going to get plenty of them when we go to the ball games and that place in Reading next to the Astor Theater. Boy, they have the tastiest Frankfurters there!!! We're going to make up for all these months we've been separated, have no fear!!!

[Wednesday] July 25th (This letter printed on 10th Mountain Division stationary)

How do you like this paper?? It's paper that some fellows had made by some printer back in Cividale and I have borrowed some. A lot has happened since I last wrote you. The order came down that we could write today but there was no guarantee about the future. Today you must excuse my handwriting if it is worse than usual because I'm writing standing up. I'm writing on the top bunk of one of the "double-decker" beds.

We're in Naples, Italy at some sort of staging area. All the men that are here, and there are lots of them, are waiting to be shipped out either directly to the Pacific or the U.S. One rumor says we'll be here 24 hours and another says we'll be here until the beginning of August. Of course, you absolutely cannot believe anything you hear. Ha! Ha! Around 6:30 this past Sunday we walked to the railroad yards where we boarded "freight" or "cattle" cars. There were 25 men in one car. On the train I was on, there were 40 cars and I was in car 38. The engine and coal car were American-made and had big U.S.A. letters on them. That trip down to Naples was an experience I'll never forget. Ha! Ha! At times we went extremely fast but then again, we just about moved at other times; and we stopped at every small town and many, many more times. It seemed that the engineer or conductor had to get a paper signed at every station. Well, we had to take turns sleeping in these cars, for not everybody could lie down comfortably. It was amazing how well I slept given the hard floor and the "rocky ride". Ha! Ha! We were given "C" rations before we left Florence for our meals on the train. We hit Leghorn at about 3 AM, on Monday and we arrived in Rome at about 5:30 PM. At the station in Rome, some Quartermaster units stationed there served the whole train with a "hot" meal. We had beef, potatoes, peas, and peaches. We didn't leave that station until 8 PM. We started again on the train at about 9:30 PM and an hour & 1/2 after we stopped and got word that we'd be delayed about 5 hours. There was some trouble ahead with regards to the tracks and repairs had to be made first. We didn't leave this area until 4:15 AM Tuesday. We arrived in Naples around noon. After we were assigned to our bunks, we went for our noon chow. I'll be doggone, the chow line here is a good half-mile in length, it takes twice as long to get your meal than it does to eat it. Ha! Ha! Looks like we'll be here until at least August 1st. When I'll be able to write again, I don't know but I was so glad to get this letter written.

[Thursday] July 26th

Dearest, simply because I've been able to write the last few days, I don't want you to start writing again. They have told us to inform those who are writing to us to discontinue since we are leaving the country and headed for the good old U.S.A. You know on one of your letters you had two three-cent stamps of that Iwo Jima[112]Edition. They are very pretty and unique stamps. Say, did Mr. Bowman ever find the culprit who was stealing gas from his car and gas pumps?? I can't see how some people can be so mean and crooked. I hope he finds the person and beats the very life from him. I have no sympathy for such people; and with the gas shortage what it is!! By the way are you people able to get enough gas?? There better not be a gas shortage when I get home. Ha! Ha! I'm not worried in the least because I'm sure Allen would give me all the gas I need, without requiring any stamps. Say, my Sweetheart, have Daddy and you carried out that plan you mentioned to me about buying one "car tax stamp" for both of you?? On the 4th of July, you had gone up home and purchased a stamp. Is that now serving both of you???

Mother tells me that you and Sister cheat terrifically at Rook. For instance, she says she asks for a small card, and then before you play you ask Sister if she can take a trick. Sister says yes and then you play the "10" of that suit. Now I just want to ask you if that is true?? If it is true, then I really believe my Wife and Sister cheat. Ha! Ha! Mother was complaining that when she asks Grandma the same question she won't answer. Yes, I believe Grandma is the only honest one of the four of you!! Well, when I get home, you are going

---

[112] This is a green 3 cent stamp showing the raising of the American flag at Iwo Jima. The public demanded a commemorative stamp, even though the US Post Office had never issued a stamp depicting a living person. On the day of issue, people were standing in line to purchase them and this stamp turned out to be one of the biggest selling stamps in Post Office history.

to be shown exactly how the game of Rook should be played. Ha! Ha! Ha!

[Friday] July 27th

Gosh, was the mailman good to me in the last few days. Last night I received a package from Mother and one from my Sweetheart and guess how many letters, thirteen!! I feel so good after reading them, only they had some sad notes in them. The letter you wrote after hearing about me coming home seemed to be a bit sad especially the first part of it. So much can happen in the next six months. I'm sure my Wife is real anxious to see her husband and I only hope that joy will "drown out" all those unpleasant thoughts. Dearest, you bit your nails again and you promised me you wouldn't. Well, you're going to have a few weeks to grow them again before I reach Berks County.

There is still nothing more definite on when we'll leave here. This morning we were given part of our PX rations. All we got was beer and cigarettes. I gave both away to other fellows. I have no use for either of them but practically all fellows consider those things the most important. Boy, I'm glad I do not have those habits. Does Walt expect to go directly to the Pacific? Gee, that's just too bad. I'm sorry for him, and his folks but the Army's policy is to send practically all service troops directly. They can feel mighty glad that he is not in a combat outfit.

Golly, but am I going to eat the Hot Dogs when that fireplace is completed!!! You must tell your parents that that was the best idea they ever had. Ha! Ha! I'll bet that after I've completed my furlough, I'll weigh a "ton"!!

[Saturday] July 28th

It remains a question as to when we'll move out. This morning our M.A.C. Officer told us it looked definite for Thursday, August 2nd but this afternoon they're saying we might board the ship on Monday. Today I received two more boxes. Honestly, I'll lose what "shape" I once had if I keep getting all these packages. The package contained a box of saltines, a jar of peanut butter, Tootsie Rolls, pineapple juice, and Lebanon bologna. You can well see what an excellent lunch it all made.

Darling, I am still so worried about your eye. The Doctor now thinks it's an allergy but had first diagnosed it as some scars from your ulcers. Gee, I'm hoping all the trouble has gone. Are those injections you are getting helping?? If it doesn't get any better seek more advice and other treatments. I'm so worried about you.

In today's "Stars & Stripes" there is an article which states that the War & Navy Dept. are expecting the war to end quicker than they had anticipated and because of that fewer men were going to be redeployed by way of the states and more men, even combat units, would go directly to the Pacific. So, everything seems to add up to us being quite fortunate to hit the states. Don't worry if you don't get any more letters, I probably won't be able to write.

[There aren't any more letters until a September 16th postcard, so Luke was furloughed home to Pennsylvania]

Furloughed to Leesport, Pennsylvania then Assigned to Camp Carson, Colorado

[Sunday] September 16th (postcard of Dolling Park, Springfield, Mo.)

It is now 11:30 AM (Central Time) and we are in Springfield, Missouri. We expect to land in Camp Carson [113] sometime tomorrow. Gee, but I dream so much about the wonderful times we had the last 30 days.

[Monday] September 17th (Western Union Telegram)

COLORADO SPRINGS, COLORADO

ARRIVED CARSON 10 AM MONDAY ADDRESS SAME AS SWIFT EXCEPT FOR CARSON. LOVE GALORE LUKE

[Monday] September 17th

This is my first letter in quite some time. When I think of the wonderful times we had the past 30 days, it makes me feel good all over. Did my Wife enjoy herself also??? Ha! Ha! Ha! I guess you're anxious to know all about our trip out here. First let me tell you that I'm writing this letter in a U.S.O. place in Colorado Springs, Colo. It is a rather nice town and I bought my wife a birthday greeting and already mailed it. I was looking around for a birthday gift but as of yet, I haven't been able to decide just what I want to get you. Please forgive me if I won't get it to you by Thursday but that would be impossible, even if I would have gotten it today.

I guess you would be very interested in all sorts of rumors I've heard since we hit Carson. I've just about heard them all.

---

[113] Camp Carson or later Fort Carson, was established in 1942 after the attack on Pearl Harbor. It was named for Army scout General "Kit" Carson who explored the West in the 1800's.

Some think we low point men will hit the Pacific before very long while others say no one will get there. The group from Pennsylvania was the first to arrive here. They expect them all back within the next 48 hours. The Camp itself reminds me a lot of Camp Swift. It has the same kind of barracks and mess hall. The part of camp we are in seems to have been vacated for many months. The grass around the building is very high and all indications point to the fact that no troops have been here for some time.

I've talked to this fellow Herb from Sunbury and his wife is going to come out here if he stays here. I've already talked to my Lt. about rooms and he says there are rooms to be had in private homes and he'd recommend some to us.

We traveled on Pullman coaches out here; not "Troop Sleepers" but regular "Compartment Pullman Sleepers". There were three in a compartment; me, Wolfe, and Miller. When we left Indiantown Gap, there were 18 coaches on the train. At Cincinnati, we dropped three and at St. Louis, we left two more off. The other thirteen coaches were 10th Mt. Division Men who came here to Camp Carson. The course went to Harrisburg on the Reading Co.[114] and then took the route of western Maryland, which traveled along the southern part of Pennsylvania. At Pittsburg, we got on the B&O[115] tracks and went down through West Virginia, came up into Ohio hitting Cincinnati. We remained on this train until St. Louis, then we got on the Frisco Lines and went through the states of Missouri, then the tip of Kansas, and headed

---

[114] Commonly called the Reading Railroad it operated in southeast Pennsylvania and neighboring states from 1924 to 1976.

[115] This stood for Baltimore and Ohio Railroad established in 1830 and then expanded into numerous branches and mergers in the 20th century.

northwest. We changed to the Santa Fe Railroad[116] in Wichita. When I say changed to another railroad, I don't mean we changed coaches, just changed to another railroad companies tracks.

Gee but I'm always thinking of the wonderful times we had together on my furlough. We are going to be so happy together in the future. Thank your parents again for that fine Doggie Roast and all those good meals I had at your place. We had such a very good time in New York and at all the baseball games we saw, didn't we??? Now, Honey, you see the Doctor and have him give you a very thorough examination and x-ray.

[Tuesday] September 18th

Darling, I came to town again this afternoon!!! Now please do not think I'm a "run around" but I did want to get my shopping done and so I did. I finally decided what to get my Dearest for her birthday; it's something that you can hardly buy in the eastern part of the country. I won't tell you what it is until I think you will have received it. Then I'll tell you exactly what it is or rather what it's made of.

I've decided to send home that $75 instead of waiting until next month. I told you they paid me at Indiantown Gap, $ 84.60. I can't in the world see how they figured my pay. According to the way I figured, they overpaid me by $50-$60. I got a money order at the post office, so let me know when you receive it.

This morning we did very little. Last night two more groups had arrived, the group from Atterbury, Indiana, and the group from Ft. Meade, Maryland. This morning a large group from Ft. Dix, New Jersey arrived. Several men haven't

---

[116] This was part of the ATSF, the Atchison, Topeka and Santa Fe Railroad, charted in 1859 which connected to Pueblo, Colorado in 1876.

come back, they remained at their redeployment center and are awaiting discharges; men with unusually high points as well as some that were 34 years and above. This fellow told me a rumor and said it came from Divisional Headquarters. He said that all men from 45 points up to the present discharge total (I think at present it is "80") would remain in the Division. Men below 45 would be screened out. According to all the latest reports about needing only 200,000 men as an occupational force, I certainly do not believe that many more men, if any, are going to be shipped to the Pacific. So, Darling, please don't worry about that.

After breakfast, I was asked to aid in setting up our Regimental Dispensary or Aid Station. We unpacked a lot of medicinal supplies and prepared to run "sick" call by tomorrow morning. We had German P.O.W.s do all the cleaning at the Dispensary. They are nice people to have around or we'd have to do all that "dirty" work. Ha! Ha! I never told you just how I come into Colorado Springs. There is a bus company which runs buses to the camp. They run every 15 minutes until 12:30 AM every night. The fare is 20 cents or you can buy 15 tokens for $1.00.

My Sweetheart, what did the Doctor say about your eye? Does my Honey feel good otherwise?? Ha! Ha!

[Wednesday] September 19th

They are finally getting things organized here at Carson. The PX has been getting in a lot of supplies lately. It's funny how ill-equipped most soldiers are after coming back from a 30-day furlough. No one seems to have any soap, toothpaste, shaving cream, and the like. I still have lots of those things which you had sent me overseas so I'm fixed, but soldiers stand in line for blocks just to purchase a cake of soap.

The rumors are still "flying" but one thing is quite certain, the 10th Mt. Division will never be broken up. It will always remain as a unit in the Regular Army in post-war years. In time only men who have volunteered for the regular army will make up the Division. I presume my wife will want me to sign up-say for another four-years, how about it?? Ha! Ha! I was talking to that fellow Herb today and he is anxious for his wife to come out but feels we should wait at least another week to find out something more definite. He said it would be nice to have you both come out together. He thinks she'll prefer to come out by train and that you could meet at Harrisburg.

Did you make an appointment with your gynecologist??? I sure hope you did. By all means, I want you to see him in case "things happen normally" in a couple of weeks. Do you understand me???? Ha! Ha! Ha! How is your eye my Darling?? If you don't think your eye is improving constantly, I wish you'd change doctors. I don't like the idea of changing glasses so frequently.

Today there wasn't much to be done. I cleaned out my barracks and duffle bag thoroughly and arranged my things. Passes are not issued now until 5:30 PM so I'm glad I went into town the last two days. Another group from Camp Grant, Illinois arrived this morning and we expect more tonight. The fellows from Grant said their engine and the first coach of their train had jumped the track on the way out but nobody was hurt.

Say, my Dearest Darling, have you been following the pennant races??? At the moment the St. Louis Cards and Chicago Cubs are playing a series that might well decide the pennant winner. I'm rooting for those cards since you'd then owe me 50 cents. Ha! Ha! I'm afraid those Detroit Tigers will win in the American League and then I'll owe you 50 cents.

You know, I still think I'm going to become an umpire. Here's a good suggestion. I'd teach school in winter and umpire in summer. You see these minor leagues don't start till May or June and stop on Labor Day. Once I get into high-class ball, I'll give up teaching-just an idea of course. Ha! Ha!

Tomorrow is my Darling's birthday and for the second straight year I'm unable to spend it with her, but I'm hoping and praying that she'll have a very happy birthday and that next year we'll spend it together.

[Thursday] September 20th

I'm so sorry I forgot to mention to the girl that your telephone number was on the Leesport exchange. You see when I wrote out the telegram and the girl read them back to me, she asked if you didn't have a telephone. I gave it to her but forgot to make mention it was the Leesport exchange. I bet you couldn't understand why they had gotten one up home and you had failed to receive one.

In today's letter, my Darling said she'd be so happy if her husband would call her up on her birthday. Well, I waited and waited to get to the booths, when I did it was 9 PM Eastern time. When I began to place the call, she said I wouldn't be able to get my call through before 9 PM Mountain time which would be 11 PM your time, or possibly even later. I'm afraid it would have been too late.

[Friday] September 21st

This afternoon at 1 PM our whole Regimental Medical Section was called together and here is what the announcement was. The War Department just sent an order through that all men who were ordered to report back to their reception or redeployment stations on the 15th of September or later would be given a 15-day furlough again. Just think of that. Almost all our men were ordered to report back on the 15th or later. There were only three camps that reported back earlier: Indiantown Gap on the 13th, Camp Atterbury, Indiana, and Ft. Dix, N.J. on the 14th. In other words, there are about 10 or 12 Medics in our Battalion from the 3 camps. All the rest reported later and now are going to get an additional 15 days furlough. By golly, it certainly seems as though luck is not with us right now. Out Regimental Surgeon said it certainly didn't seem fair to those of us who couldn't go home. Then I asked him if we men who weren't able to go home would get first preference on furloughs when other regular ones would be given and he said "yes". In the meantime, our Regimental Commanding Officer said there would not be much for us to do. It's beginning to seem to me that the Division will never assemble as a unit. I believe they don't know exactly what to do with all these men.

Has Sarah made up her mind as to whether she'll come out here? That really would be wonderful if you could come with her. Would she drive out? Why don't you approach her in the matter? She might decide to if you would go along. Dearest, by now you should also have received your birthday gift. You can hardly buy a kind of metal bracelet like that in the East. It is made in Mexico and it's known as Mexican Silver. The only thing I did not like about it is that those interlocking claps seem to be too far apart. If they are you could maybe close them with "pliers". Gee, I hope you'll enjoy it.

I'm so glad to hear that the Doctor thinks your eye looks so good. Did he mention anything about getting new glasses? Did my Honey Darling eat too much on her birthday?? Gee, I hope not but I hope she had a very happy and joyous day. She deserves the best. Love Galore Luke

[Saturday] September 22nd

It is 8:20 back home and I guess my Honey is home by now, probably writing to her husband. I often like to think of the exact thing that my wife is doing. It makes me feel so close to her. What kind of weather are you having? Sister writes that they are having the "stoker" [117] going at a pretty good clip up home. Is it getting cool? Here in Colorado, it has gotten quite a lot warmer.

Those men who were eligible for another 15 days left this afternoon. So there aren't many of us Medics left. Ha! Ha! This morning the whole 85th Regiment was addressed by the Regimental Commander. He claims that too many men who go on pass do not "dress" properly; they fail to wear their "combat jacket" when wearing their O.D.s. He warned us that if we did not improve there would be no more passes given. Now that we're back in the garrison the "army" is bearing down "again". Ha! Ha! This morning our 1st Sergeant told the rest of us that Major General Hays, our Divisional Commander, was making an effort to get the rest of us an additional 15 days also. Gee, it's so hard to decide now whether you should come out here.

This morning I inquired from our Regimental C.O. when and where church services would be held. While talking he asked me if I'd like a new job. The mail clerk who had charge of all the mail for the Medics in the 85th Regiment has over seventy points and therefore will soon be getting out of the Army. He said I could have the job if I want it. The job calls for a Corporal Technician and I'd be attached to the Regimental Medical Section instead of the 3rd Battalion. I guess I'd be suited for the job so I'll probably take it.

---

[117] This was a mechanical device that fed coal into the furnace which saved the home owner from doing it manually.

Sweetheart, I'm so afraid you're not happy and that makes me feel bad. Please do not let your loneliness make you down-hearted. When you feel like that just remember all the things that we can be grateful and happy for and remember there is always a silver lining in every cloud. Remember that portion of scripture that goes something to this effect, "If God is for you who can be against you".

I'm seeing quite a lot of this fellow Briggs from Philadelphia. The 2nd Battalion Medical Station is right next to ours so we see each other every day. He's one fellow I know of who has fewer points than I do.

[Sunday] September 23rd

I can easily see that my Darling was disappointed because she didn't get a phone call from her hubby on Thursday night. Please forgive me, my Dear, I really made an effort but the long delay and the two hours difference in time would have caused it to get too late. I'll try to get a phone call through some time near future.

In the "day room" which is just a few buildings away from our barracks they have a ping pong table and this fellow Briggs wants me to play him some time. He's pretty good and he'll probably beat the living "daylights" out of me. Ha! Ha! But it will give me something to do. He also asked me to go into Colorado Springs tonight and go to church with him. It depends on how I feel. The buses going into town are usually so full and I'd think especially so on Sunday night. This morning I read the Sunday paper. The main paper here is the "Denver Post" and the one thing I don't like about it is it's a Republican paper. Ha! Ha! Speaking of papers, is the "Eagle" and "Times" printers still on strike?? Boy and now with the World Series coming up and no Reading Times. Is my Darling still following the baseball leagues? Today a week the regular season closes and the World Series[118] starts. Well, I'm quite sure the Detroit Tigers will win the American League pennant.

Darling, you asked about our barracks!!! The buildings we live in here are the same as at Swift and Indiantown Gap. They are two-story barracks and painted that cream color. My bunk is on the second floor. There are very few men in the building. About 35 men can sleep on one floor and there are only five of us, so you can see how empty it is. We eat as we did at Barkeley, family-style. Everything is just put on the table and you help yourself. Since so many men are on furlough, they had an excess of food. I had three "blocks" of ice cream for dessert.

[Monday] September 24th

I'm wondering if my Dearest heard what I did this morning. First, I heard it as a rumor but then later this morning Briggs told me he heard it announced over the radio. They've dropped the number of points for men not going overseas to 36. In other words, any soldier with 36 or more points as of September 2nd will not go overseas. If that is true that just lets me in. I have either 36 or 37 but I'm absolutely sure of 36 points so Honey Bunch you don't have to worry about your hubby going to Japan. I had a hunch anyway that I wasn't going over but there isn't a thing to worry about. If I take this Regimental mail clerk job, I'd surely remain in the Division too.

I did go to church with Briggs last night. We left here about 6:30 and got to town about 7, looked up the church directory, and saw that the "First Baptist Church" had services at 7:30 and the church was not far from the USO so

---

[118] Although controversial, baseball was kept going during the war years since it seemed to serve as a morale booster for the American people.

we decide to go there. They had a very fine service. If and when you come out here, we'll have to visit that church.

It still seems to be quite a strong rumor that we fellows that are here will receive furloughs soon after the men return. Nothing is definite. I don't want you to come until after you see the Doctor, if necessary, then I'll probably know more by that time. Please make an appointment with the Doctor because things are going to start rolling and once they start, there is no telling when they'll stop. Ha! Ha! It's usually the guess that when "they" start coming they come pretty easy. Then watch out!!!!! We'll see what develops in the next couple of weeks.

This morning there wasn't anything to be done. I went over to the "office" the mail clerk has and he told me all his duties and the like, in case I take the job. I went to the Regimental Post Office; saw where to pick up the mail. I enjoy working with mail but I'd be moved out of the 3rd Battalion and put in the Regimental Medical Station.

Yes, my Sweetheart, I too am convinced now that "Flush" is worth every bit of the $25.00. She is a very fine dog and she likes me so much, doesn't she? I'm positive now that when we have a home of our own, we'll have a dog and preferably a "cocker", how about it???

[Tuesday] September 25th

Well, I heard some news today that I'm sure you'll be "tickled" to hear. We fellows are definitely going to get furloughed in about a week. Now I was going to send a telegram from camp here for some money but I've been told that they are lined up for blocks at the telegraph office, so I'll have you go to town this evening and send the telegram from Western Union. I'm sure we won't leave before today a week so I feel as though sending me a money order would be O.K.

I guess the Army doesn't know what to do with us fellows so they let us spend the time at home until we get our discharge. If only I'd be stationed at a camp closer to Pennsylvania then the traveling expenses would not be an item. Exactly what the fare is, I don't know. They say anywhere from $38 to $50 round trip, so I'm sure if you send me $50 it will be sufficient. You can send it by Western Union or get a money order and send it airmail. I wish now I wouldn't have sent you that $75 but I expected to stay here or be moved at Government expense. There's talk that we'll get another 45-day furlough and I possibly might be home for Christmas. Oh, happy day!!!! Who said I wasn't getting any breaks! Ha! Ha!

Have the papers gone to press yet??? Boy, they better would have until I get home or I'll tell those printers what I think of them. Ha! Ha! Don't worry; I guess my bark is louder than my bite!!! Have you made an appointment with your gynecologist??? Gee, I hope so because we have to get things rolling one of these months!!

[Wednesday] September 26th

I just got back from the Signal Office that is located here on the post and received a Western Union money order of $60.00. I must go into town to get it cashed. Gosh, the place was so crowded. I bet there were more than 50 men there waiting for money to arrive by telegram. I sent a night letter, which is cheaper and the message was not urgent enough to have to be delivered before this morning. What time did you receive the telegram? I hope it was before 8 AM so you could have taken the money right with you. After I sent the telegram, I went to the Railroad Station at Colorado Springs and got the information on trains leaving town. On the fastest train you'll need a reservation and not knowing what day I'll get my furloughed, I can't make a reservation. I'll just get the first train out unless I can catch a bus for Denver first. I can catch a train there and there are many more and faster trains leaving from there. We are allowed three days of traveling time each way. Here's some more news. Those future 45-day furloughs have been temporarily canceled. All I'm hoping for is that I'll be able to come home for Christmas. A fellow couldn't ask for more.

Dearest, I'm very glad to see that you're interested in getting more insurance. I think insurance is a wonderful thing and I'm sure we can meet those increased payments on the policies you are thinking about. Since I expect to be home in a rather short time why not let things go until then and we'll talk things over when I get back.

[Thursday] September 27th

So, my Dearest knows that the points have been dropped to 36 for overseas duty. I'm sure that I have 36 or 37. You know they only had me down for 29 as of May 12th. Well, we got seven more up until V-J Day.

I'm so glad you like your birthday gift. Yes, they claimed it's real Mexican Silver. I, of course, am no authority on that kind of metal but I believe it is quite a bit different than anything you can buy at home. Now, I presume, you've sent me back $60 of that $75 I sent you. I'm sorry that I had to ask for money but I didn't have nearly enough to come home.

So, you can't see the gynecologist until November 5th?? Boy, he really must be busy!! Well, you'll go to him then if nothing "develops" in the meantime. Ha! Ha! Ha! Your hubby will be home in the meantime and one never knows!! If you would have known he was filled up that much you could have called much earlier. Well, you surely are going to see him this time if nothing "happens" in the meantime.

So, my Sweetheart is traveling on one of those new buses. Say but I'll bet they are nice! When I come home, I think we'll have to travel on them just for curiosity's sake. You know I'm a great fellow when it comes to something like that. Ha! Ha! I guess you think sometimes that you've married one funny man. Does my Sweetheart want to bet on the World Series??? You pick the team you want and we'll bet $1, $2, $3, $4, or $5. It looks like Chicago and Detroit.

[Friday] September 28th

This morning the temperature was reported as being 25 degrees and there was some snow on the ground too. Imagine, snow on Sept. 28th. We could see quite a bit of snow on the mountain ranges in the distance. I guess we'll have to move out to Colorado since I enjoy snow so much, how about it??

Well, the way things look I have that mail clerk job wrapped up in a bag whether I want it or not. I took care of all the mail again this morning; I'm doing the job now already and believe me, that's a job I know how to handle. Ha! Ha!

That fellow Herb and I went into town to cash our money orders and ended up running all over town trying to find the best train schedule. Of course, we must try and find out just what day we are getting furloughed, that's important, you know. Ha! Ha! This fellow Herb is really a nice guy. I didn't get to know him too well because in combat he worked the Aid Station. He writes to his wife every day too. He wrote and told his wife about you and the fact that you two could come out together and she wrote back she was anxious to meet you.

Say, my Darling is getting to be an expert driver now that she can even drive through water and not "stall" the motor. Whenever you have to drive through fairly deep water always go very slowly and shift into second or even "low" gear so you are sure you won't have to change gears and thereby "stall" the car. How does the Chevy work?? I hope she doesn't get "hot" anymore.

[Saturday] September 29th

You know Ruth Dear, I never got an opportunity to make a phone call. Whenever I get the chance the delay was so long that it would be late in the night until you'd receive it. You asked me if I'd rather stay in Camp Carson than any other camp in the States??? It's a nice place but one thing is that it's too far from Berks County.

Our Regimental Surgeon told us that on Monday about 700 recruits are coming here as replacements in the 10th Mt. Division. It looks like I'll be stationed here permanently. Ruth Darling, Herb has 51 points as of V-J Day.

Darling, one of the nicest things about traveling is changing from one train or bus to another and you say that's what you don't like. I enjoy changing. You wouldn't have to worry about not getting on the right train, it's very simple. I thought my Sweetheart never took aspirins, but she did now. Well, I'm very "frank" with you; I don't like you to use them either. I've more or less made up my mind that I won't use them anymore. They aren't good for a person's heart and after all, I can stand a little pain from a headache. Glad to hear that you and Sister had a milkshake together last night.

Now you must be sure and listen to the World Series whenever you possibly can. Pick a team and I'll pick the other. They are so evenly matched I can't be sure which will win. I just heard the Cubs clinched the pennant.

Yes, Ruth, a Corporal receives about $15 or $20 a month more than a Pfc. so naturally, it's good that I become a Corporal Technician with the mail clerk job.

[There are no further letters until October 22nd so it seems Luke got his furlough home soon after the 29th of September]

[Monday] October 22nd (aboard Jeffersonian-mailed from St Louis)

Here I go again writing to my Darling Wife. I left her yesterday at 5:15 PM, called her at 9 PM, and now I'm writing at 7:30 AM. The train left Harrisburg about 20 minutes late and now she's running about 50 minutes behind schedule.

Gee whiz, but we had such a wonderful time again, didn't we? I can't wait until I receive that next furlough.

[Tuesday] October 23rd

I arrived at Colorado Springs at about 8:30 AM. Herb and I had something to eat then we went out to Camp and what I have to say to you now will really be of interest I'm sure. It came as a shock to me but it goes to show, you never can be sure of anything in the Army. As the bus approached the part of the camp that houses the 10th Mt Division, we remarked that there seemed to be so few men around. The fellow in front of us turned around and asked us if we didn't know that the Division was being deactivated. Yes, about a week ago the order came down from Washington that this Division will be broken up. They claim they are going to send us to different units according to the number of points we have. One rumor says men with 36 to 50 pts. will be sent to Camp Swift, Texas. Captain Goffrey told me that the Medics would be the last group to leave, probably around the 11th of November. Nothing more has been said about those 45-day furloughs. I'm glad that we decided that you would not come along because you'd probably want to go home when I'm moved. After all, I'd move on an Army order and you couldn't come with me.

Well, I took over the mail clerk's job officially today. Captain Goffrey (our Regimental Surgeon) told me that I should bring up to date all the records of the men as to their addresses so that they can all be turned in when other records go in. There is a lot of work to that and the former clerk didn't have everything up to par. So now you can rest assured that I have plenty to do. One of the mail clerks at the Regimental Post Office told me that all unit mail clerks would be declared essential men and would remain here after all the men from their outfit had left to re-route all mail that will come in. I don't know whether I'm coming or going. Ha! Ha!

We arrived in St. Louis about 2:30 on Monday and then got in line to board the "Colorado Eagle"[119] and guess what, Herb and I didn't even get a seat. We stood from 4:15 until 9:30 PM. At that time, we arrived in Kansas City and it so happened that a couple of sailors got off, we sat down and fell asleep. Ha! Ha!

Boy oh boy, it's cold here!! It was snowing when we got off the train and snowed off and on most of the day. There is a terrifically strong wind blowing and it is very cold.

(Enclosed in this letter is a newspaper clipping entitled:
"10TH MOUNTAIN DIVISION BEING DEACTIVATED"
Famed Infantry Outfit Mustering Out at Camp Carson

---

[119] This passenger train was operated by the Missouri Railroad until 1964, traveling between St. Louis and Denver. A picture of it shows a streamlined engine, mostly dark blue with a cream and silver design across the sides with the lower edge outlined in yellow. There is a wing spread eagle in chrome across the nose of the engine.

Colorado Springs, Oct 23- The famous Tenth Infantry Mountain Division which bulked large in the final Allied campaign in Italy, is being deactivated at Camp Carson, the others being sent to various centers for discharge. Some 1200 have been discharged here and many others will be released soon. Low-point men not eligible for discharge are being sent to other centers pending release.

After its activation in July 1943, the Tenth trained at Camp Hale, near Leadville, it was the only mountain division in the army.

The division's instructors were famous skiers, rock climbers, and guides from all sections of the country. The men underwent arduous training in mountain climbing, physical aid, and lived in arctic tents.

It was the first division to enter the Po Valley in Italy and the first to cross the Po River. In four months of combat, approximately 1,000 were killed and more than 3,000 wounded.)

[Wednesday] October 24th

The weather has taken a turn again and the temperature has gone up. The sun is very warm and we have the doors and windows of the barracks open, but it was cold during the night. I'm really trying to reduce. Yesterday I missed the evening meal and I think I'll do the same today.

The mail goes out at 8:30, by that we unit mail clerks must have all our mail down at the Regimental Post Office by that time. At 11:00 I went down and received the incoming mail. There are still some men who have not come back and whose mail I'm holding, but I've made up my mind-if they soon don't return, I'm going to return their mail to the sender. You see some men were held at their reception centers awaiting discharge. They never have sent us their home address and so I have no choice but to return their mail. I came over here to my "room" I have in one corner of our supply building. There is a table here and it is nice to write but yesterday it was too cool since there is no fire in the room.

This noon an announcement was made in the mess hall that all men with less than 50 points would remain close to their barracks because an official order is supposed to be forthcoming. I haven't heard any more about the mail clerks staying here but that might be true.

This morning we turned in to the supply room a list of clothing shortages. I'm hoping to get another O.D. shirt. They still don't have my size. Well, if I lose a little weight, I'll be able to wear a 15 1/2 collar and that size they have.

You know I've done a terrible thing. I've worried about it quite a bit. You know the key that unlocks the "lock" on the garage door of the garage up home; well, I forgot to leave it at home. I discovered it in my pocket on the way to Harrisburg. I wanted to mention it when I called on Sunday but it slipped my mind. I planned to send it home in a letter and guess what happened- I lost it! I've looked and looked and still can't find it and I believe it was the only key they had. If I can't find it, I presume the only thing they can do is "break" the lock. Is my Honey mad at me????

Are you having those drops put in your eye regularly this week?? I'm so anxious to hear what the Doctor has to say about your eye. Be sure and tell him the whole thing; and also your GYN Doctor. Gosh, if you don't feel in the least bit "sick" by Monday night I'd tell him about it. I can hardly wait to see how all these things turn out.

[Thursday] October 25th

The mail is getting heavier since most of the fellows are returning from their furloughs. With papers and packages plus letters, I'm getting so much I'll soon have to get a "jeep" to get my mail. Ha! Ha! Ha!

Nothing materialized yesterday as to any official order. Last night I spoke to a fellow from I Company and he said that today he's leaving for Camp Swift, Texas. He thinks about 1000 men from the regiment are leaving with him and he believes they all have 44 and fewer points and he also thinks that all with 35 and less are included. I also learned that one Medic from our regiment will be transferred to Fort Bliss, Texas. He's the only one from our outfit so far that is being moved. There have been strong rumors that the whole Medical Detachment would be moved as a unit, regardless of points, to some hospital.

How does my Darling feel about me leaving here? Is she sad or glad?? The only thing I don't like is the uncertainty of the next furlough. As soon as I hit my new camp, I'm due this furlough time, and by gosh I'm going to try as hard as possible to get it over Christmas. Gee it would be wonderful to be home over Christmas.

[Friday] October 26th

As soon as I picked up the mail at 11 AM I went through all of it at the Regimental Post Office and looked for my mail. Sister's letter was postmarked 9:30 PM on Wednesday so you see that it made excellent time. It's funny how some letters make such excellent time while others take 4-5 days. I have gotten everything pretty well under control now so things run much more smoothly. This afternoon I came over to my "office" and was ready to start my letters when our Section

Sgt. came in and asked me to umpire a softball game. I told him I wanted to write but he insisted that I do it.

This evening there is going to be a dinner for the whole Regimental Medical Detachment at some hotel in Manitou Springs, about 6-7 miles from Colorado Springs. Transportation will be furnished and all you want to eat. I'm quite sure I won't go. I don't feel very much like attending such affairs.

Around noon today a clerk from our Regimental Personnel Office came into the barracks and said that one of his battle stars had been taken away from him because he was in the hospital during the whole push through the Po Valley and that as a result, he only had 33 points (with that star he'd have 38). He said that as a result of having only 33 he'd be leaving here within a few days, probably to Camp Swift. Yes, they are really getting men with 35 and fewer points out of here. The rumor has it that they are going to the South Pacific to relieve high point men. Boy, I'm just in "safe" territory with my 36 points.

So, you've worked the first three days of this week!! I certainly believe that now you'll work every day this week. I believe you'd rather do that than look for another place to work, wouldn't you?? You've always said you'd rather be kept busy than have a lot of time on your hands, even if Anita does give you more work than the other girls. I wouldn't kick. The less said the better. But Honey, if you hate it too much why just stop. All the money in the world isn't worth that much.

I can easily see by the letters my Darling wrote me after finding out about my 15-day furlough that she had her heart set on coming out here with me. She would have enjoyed very much to drive out too, wouldn't she?? Now she didn't get her wish!! My only hope is that I'm closer to Pennsylvania and get a furlough over Christmas, even if it is only a short one.

[Saturday] October 27th

You asked me in your letter how I enjoy being a mail clerk? Well, I like it all right except that with the Division being broken up it will mean more work for one. It doesn't matter too much what a fellow does in the Army as long as he has to be in the "thing" anyway. Ha! Ha!

On the way to my barracks, I heard a "football broadcast" on a radio in the barracks occupied by the Medics of 1st Battalion, so I stopped in to hear the game for a few minutes. While there, the Regimental Clerk for the personnel office told me that my Class B allotment had been discontinued for July and August. Class B allotment is your "bond" allotment. He said they made the error at my reception center by paying me the money instead of figuring the allotment. He said, however, that I'd be getting the bonds again starting with September. That at least, partially, accounts for all that money I received at Indiantown Gap. The clerk also told me an interesting thing. He said that I was officially declared essential and that I'd remain here at Camp until the whole Division was moved out, not only until all the Medics leave. I still think I should be out of here by Dec. 1st. Being essential can turn out to be either good or bad, in case the Division takes longer to break up, I might be stuck here too long and won't get a chance to get my furlough from my new camp in time for Christmas. I believe that any man who is declared essential will be given his preference as to what camp he wants to go to. If that would be the case, I'd ask for Indiantown Gap.

Here's something!! You know our First Sgt. asked me when I got back on Tuesday as to whether I received notice officially that I was a T/5; I said no. He said he'd check the matter right away. Well, here's what they told me now. My rating was acted upon and it passed Regimental Headquarters O.K. but when it reached Divisional Headquarters, they sent down an order that no more ratings would be given. They were "frozen" on September 30th and my rating went in on October 1st. Hereafter telling me that I already had it!!! He said my Capt. is going further. He is going to the Adjutant General Office personally and feels he'll be able to make it official. In the meantime, I'm a Corporal in authority and name but most important of all not financially. What a Break!!!

Dearest, you must go roller-skating with those girls. I know you enjoy that sport and it does you good to have some entertainment. You do not get out enough. I know my Honey will behave alright.

[Sunday] October 28th

I presume Mother, Father, and Grandma were glad to see you after not seeing you since Sunday. Dearest, you must not be afraid to drive the car at night!! Gosh, there isn't anything to it!!! Certainly, sooner or later you'll have to do a lot of driving at night. Aren't you going to help me drive when you go with me to camp after my next furlough??? Or did you expect me to do all the driving??? Ha! Ha! Ha! I knew my wife wouldn't have any trouble getting out of the city. It's all in your mind. How did you leave the city? Did you go out 4th St.?? Yes, I too must "pat" you on the back for being such a good driver. Ha! Ha! Ha!

You asked me in a letter whether I'd be "broke" if I'd give up my mail clerk job. I'm not at all together positive on that score but I believe I would be in this case, unless your officer would transfer you to another job that called for the same rating. As a rule, however, any technician's rating is more secure than other ratings. Of course, if you are insubordinate you can be "busted". Yes, the only thing a rating is good for is the extra money that a fellow gets.

[Monday] October 29th

The way things look right now, the Medical Detachment will be broken up the same as the other line companies (Infantrymen). This morning I was told by the personnel clerk that men with 50- 59 points are going to be transferred to the "Service Command" here at Camp Carson and then will be shipped to some other camps as "Military Police" (M.P.s). Of course, all men with 60 to 70 points will be getting discharged within the next month.

Gee but I so wish I knew how my Darling feels at this very moment. Tonight at 9:15, I believe, she has her appointment with her GYN. Does my Sweetheart feel as though she is going to get "sick" or is she "sick" already or just how does she feel??? I can hardly wait until I receive your letters of this week.

Did Anita tell you not to come in today?? Gee, I wish my Dearest would go to a place to work where she thinks she'll like it. If my Darling wants to get a job somewhere else that's perfectly alright, and if she doesn't want to that's alright also. You tell me in your letter that if you'd known I'd be home in a couple of weeks you wouldn't even bother getting a job! Well, I wouldn't count on me being home in a couple of weeks. But Honey, please, please do not worry about a single thing especially our finances.

Why in the world didn't you go along with your Aunts and Mary to see Duffy's Tavern?? I'm sure you would have enjoyed it. You had told me you would like to see it. Did you go rollerskating with those girls yet??? Now I'm ordering you to go to these entertainments. Please be a good girl and listen to your husband. Are you sure you're reading "nice" books just now? Boy, I'm surprised at the "trash" you were reading!!! My Wife is so "sexy", much more so than her husband is. Ha! Ha! Ha!

[Tuesday] October 30th

Oh my, but I've been thinking about you so very much the last 24 hours. Last night you went to the Doctor and also this morning. Did you tell the Dr. that we were together a few times??? Did he examine you, that is, would whatever he did cause you to get sick if beforehand you wouldn't have???

Well, this morning when I got the mail there was a letter from Sister. She said Daddy fell again and broke the card table. I can't help but pity Daddy because he is so helpless and then to all the work and worriment it causes Mother and Sister. Sister thinks he hurt his head pretty badly when he fell. I hope it's not serious. But there is so little that can be done, we just can't let it worry us. That's the way life is.

My Sweetheart asked me a funny question in one of her letters last week. She asks if my bed here was as good as the one back home and how it feels to be back in the Army after 19 days as a civilian? Well, here's my answer: anyone who wants to exchange his civilian status for my Army life, I'll gladly trade with him.

Yes, I guess you could easily tell that the card I sent you was written on the train. It rocks just enough to make your penmanship almost resemble "scribbling". It really is hard to write on the train.

Nothing more has been said about my T/5 rating and I'm soon going to speak to my Capt. about it. The TO (Army regulations) call for a rating for the mail clerk, all the others always had one, and now with this work of straightening out the records and the like and not getting the extra money would really "rile" me. I guess you think your hubby is angry now. Ha! Ha! He's not that mad though!!!!

Say, I bet the kitchen over home looks nice. Yes, Mama does a good job at such things. Anything having to do with painting, carpentry and the like, she is very good at and also sewing. You must thank her again for laundering my shirts. That was very nice of her.

I like that violet ink, I noticed it in the first letter I received from you. It is much more outstanding on white paper than it is on the blue. You've used about every color now but green.

[Wednesday] October 31st

Are you out celebrating Halloween this evening?? I haven't seen much of Halloween here in camp. It's just another day. I remember when we were in High School, we had Halloween parties every year. I wonder if they still have them? They also had a big parade up in Hamburg during the Halloween season. Wasn't that called the King Frost Carnival?? I think we were up there one time, weren't we??

I am surprised that we are having such mild weather the last week of October. Gee whiz, there are only two more months and 1945 will be history. Well, I hope that the future years will be more enjoyable than this one has been; and yet, while we were separated the greater part of the year, we still are quite lucky that we are all alive and well. Let's only pray that we will soon be together for good.

I was sorry to hear that you are not going to work at your place anymore. I know you didn't like the girls but there were a lot of things that were all right. For one, you liked the hours pretty well and you got to know the customers, too. But please, my Sweetheart, don't worry in the least about that. I'm so anxious to hear whether you started working at the new beauty shop. Isn't that place pretty far up on Penn Street?? Did you go to see the girl who manages the Glo-Ray beauty shop??

This morning orders came through for three of the Medics to leave tomorrow. All three have some 50 points. They are all going to the "Service Command Unit" (Military Police) here at Camp Carson. I believe that before the week is over practically all 50 to 59 pt. men will be leaving.

So, Earl is home and discharged!! How does he look in civilian clothes? I'll bet Rachael is so happy she doesn't know what to do. So, Russell also is discharged!!! Gee, he's been in the Army for such a long time. My Honey thinks her hubby should get his civilian suits tailored so that he can slip right into them when he gets home. You know what?? You're making me real, real anxious!!! Gosh, it seems so long since I've had on a civilian suit that I won't know what it feels like. Ha! Ha! Ha!

Did my Sweetheart get "sick" before Monday night? I hope not, but I'll have to wait until I get your letter tomorrow to find out.

[Thursday] November 1st

The weather has gotten a bit colder today. The wind is really strong. It blows you right off your feet if you don't watch yourself. Ha! Ha!

Well, more rumors are flying around and I don't believe any of them. They seem too fantastic to be true. This morning I was talking to our supply Sgt. and he was also declared essential. Well, he thinks we men will probably get a good break from it all. He thinks that we fellows might get a discharge before too long or be sent to our reception centers, which in my case would be Indiantown Gap. Another rumor is that Medics with 36 to 50 pts. are going to be assigned to hospital ships that are bringing back wounded veterans from Europe and the South Pacific. Every hour you hear something different and yet no one knows anything.

Nothing more has been said to me about my rating and I am honestly beginning to believe that once again I'm going to be left out. They all want me to have it but the fact that Division "froze" all ratings is where the catch comes in.

Is my Sweetheart working at the new shop now??? Yes, it certainly didn't take long to get another place to work, did it? Well, I guess the girl knew you were a good operator and made room for you.

I'm so anxious to receive the letter you wrote on Tuesday to see what the Doctor had to say. I'm almost positive you will not have gotten "sick" before Monday night if you weren't at noon yet. I can hardly wait to hear what Dr. B says about your eye. I'm sure he'll be able to correct anything that might be the matter.

I've been helping our Supply Sgt. part of the afternoon. We were issued quite a bit more equipment. I got another O.D. shirt and I've got in for another pair of pants. It helps when you know the Supply Sgt. Ha! Ha! They gave us some heavy underwear also.

Gee, but I'm in love. I wish you knew how much I love you.

[Friday] November 2nd

Dearest, it hurts me terribly to hear how painful that examination was with your gynecologist. Oh, if only I could have been there to help you. I'm glad if he finds everything O.K. Of course, it doesn't make me feel good to know that it's now my fault, but I always felt as though it couldn't be anything the matter with my Sweetheart. I'd rather go out and work in a "labor gang" if that would help me get more cells. Did the Doctor say anything as to how a fellow can receive more cells??? Gee, I can't see why I should have less than any other fellow. Did you have your "period" by this time??? In case you had been pregnant would what he did have spoiled everything?? Oh my, but I feel so sorry for my Darling for what she went through.

So, you think Dr. B. gave you a good examination?? Is there nothing that he can do to rid you of that tissue?? Did you tell him you thought your sight was a bit impaired?? I'm glad you have faith in him. How much did he charge you?? Doesn't he want to see you again to see if more tissue has disappeared?

Well, today my Darling is going to work at the new place again. I'm sure she'll like everything but those hours. That gets you home late every night. If I were you, I'd use the Chevy to go back and forth to work. You could be home an hour earlier every day and it won't cost any more. You're paying $3.50 for 10 round trips and you can make more than 10 round trips on $3.00 worth of gas.

Well, this morning I spoke to my Captain. He spoke very highly of me but they absolutely refuse to grant me my increased rating. He should have a Major's rating but he too wasn't granted it. I'll never believe a thing I'm told in this man's Army because it's always going to be changed anyway. So, I'm definitely not a Corporal except in the work I'm doing and my authority but the most important thing -the extra money, I'm not getting.

[Saturday] November 3rd

I attended to my mail business as usual this morning. Yes, I certainly do get the "raw" deals. This mail job is all right but I certainly would never have taken the responsibility if I'd have known I would not get extra money. Now that I have it the First Sgt. and my Captain insists I keep it. More work but no more money!!! Ha! Ha! Oh well, what's money anyway!! How about it???

On Monday, Herb will leave us. About 6 or 10 Medics are leaving at the beginning of the next week and Herb is one of them. He's going to a hospital as an M.P. I believe, in Springfield, MO. Some of the others are going to a camp in Kansas and one, I think, is going to Minnesota. Boy, there will be work now for me in straightening out each man's record and forwarding his mail.

There are very strong rumors that men with 36-39 points will be transferred to the 75th Field Artillery which is located here at Camp Carson. It, however, also is going to be deactivated and turned into a "truck battalion" and then be sent to Camp Gruber, Oklahoma.

Before starting your letter, I heard the latter part of the Navy-Notre Dame football game. It was a real "thriller" and ended in a 6-6 tie. It was played before 80,000 people in Cleveland.

Say, wouldn't that be something if they built a diner across the street from us!! I'll bet we'd have all the hamburgers and French fries we could eat. Gosh, just talking about it makes my mouth water. Ha! Ha!

Dr. B. certainly didn't charge you much for the examination he gave you, did he? I'm only hoping your eye will continue to get better. Dearest, do you still feel sore?? Do you have your "period" now or is the womb bleeding because he cut it!!?? Oh, if I were only home to help my Honey Bunch.

[Sunday] November 4th

Dearest, guess what, in a very short time I'll be talking to my Honey Bunch. I came into Colorado Springs and here at the USO, they have a telephone operator who puts in the call for you. In the letter I received from you yesterday, you seemed so anxious that I call you up. You said you'd be up home all afternoon so I put the call in for 23-R2. I only hope it will come through before 7:30 E.S.T. because you'll be going to church then. The operator said she didn't think the delay would be so very long. It's some $2.00 for 3 minutes. I reversed the charges; I hope you won't mind. You and the folks up at home can fight it out as to who pays the bill. Ha! Ha! In the meantime, while I'm waiting for the call to come through, I'm writing to my Sweetheart.

Gee, but it's a lovely day here in Colorado. The sun is hot. As soon as the sun goes down however it gets quite chilly but in the middle of the day, it is quite warm. There isn't a cloud in the sky.

Honey Dear, I was a bad boy!! I forgot to tell you something in yesterday's letter. We got paid. I received $36.08. I can't figure out how I got so much money if I only received Pfc. wages. Either they didn't take my bond allotment out again or they gave me too much money. I receive between $16 & $17 a month as a Pfc. when $18.75 is taken out and that is enough for me a month. If you'd rather have the money, I'll cut the bonds out and send you $20.00 a month but I don't need all that money when I'm in the Army.

[3:55 PM]

Gosh, alive, I just got finished talking to my Dearest Wife and folks. Man, did that make me feel good. Oh my, but I was so glad to talk to you. Gee, I only hope the bill wasn't too much. Did my Darling enjoy hearing her hubby's voice?? It really is wonderful. You're almost 2000 miles away and we talked to each other. That is something, isn't it??? Gosh, I'm thinking of so many things that I had wanted to say and I didn't think of them when I was on the phone.

So, you're playing Rook at this particular time, are you?? Gee, I hope my Honey is having a good time at the moment. Are you happy my Sweetheart?? Oh my, but I love you so very, very much. You deserve the very best of everything in all the world.

[Monday] November 5th

I'm so anxious to hear how my Darling liked her first day's work at the Glo-Ray?? I'm so glad you were able to make the 5:30 bus on Friday and Saturday. If I understand you correctly, you said that whenever you're not busy you'll be able to catch that bus and if you're busy you'll work until 6:00 and then catch the 7 PM bus. Well, that doesn't sound bad at all. I only hope my Sweetheart likes her work all right. Now if you don't, you just quit, understand???

Well, this afternoon about 10 Medics are leaving and this morning at 10:30 an order came through for five more, and they left already at 11 AM. They are really starting to move them out. They claim that the whole camp will be closed by Nov. 30th. Like Camp Barkeley the whole place will close.

I wouldn't think about me coming to my reception center too much because I don't believe that will happen. I don't think anything that good could happen to me. Ha! Ha! All I'm hoping for is that I move at least closer to home. I don't want to go further west.

Yes, my Dear, I guess I must get a few of my suits altered before I can wear them; the new one and my second newest for sure. Maybe those older suits will fit me pretty well now.

Boy, will I feel good when I can put on a civilian suit. It's nice to think about, isn't it???

Say, that surprises me about Frank quitting at Carpenter Steel. Well, for 30 cents an hour more it's worth considering. Of course, his job might not be as permanent at Berks Engineering as it was at Carpenter. So, Uncle Eddie also quit at Carpenter. Well, work down there won't be so good I'm afraid, but yet it's always nice to know a job is waiting for you. They've always treated me pretty well. Yes, taking that course in spectroscopy may mean a lot to me.

Dearest, now please forget about not writing to me last Sunday two weeks ago. I should never have expected one. You are so very, very faithful to me.

[Tuesday] November 6th

I received Friday's letter and you had just completed your first day's work at your beauty shop. Did you mean there are only three of you working there? The manager and a man, besides you? Did the other girl quit??? So, my Honey Bunch is working with a "man"!! As soon as I got your letter, I thought I'd "kid" you about that!! Ha! Ha! I guess you'll soon forget about your hubby out here in Colorado!!

As usual, I attend to my mail business. I'm getting quite a bit of mail on hand. I really will have a headache until the thing is straightened out. Ha! Ha! We had an inspection of uniforms this morning. You've got to be shaved smoothly and your hair cut short enough. I was well shaven but the 1st Sgt. said I'd better get a haircut before tomorrow.

Our First Sgt. told us that all men 50-59 pts. who have yet been transferred will be declared surplus and discharged within a few days. Up until this week, men were discharged right from this camp but they've closed that part of the camp and now men will return to their reception centers to be discharged.

Today is election day and I'm hoping my Honey will go up to vote. You encourage your parents to go too. I'm anxious to see how the returns come in. The Democrats will easily carry the country. I'm interested in our township elections for the school director.

Say, I've got some news for you. I walked down to the PX last evening, saw a scale, stepped on it, and guess what I weigh-203 lbs. and I had a field jacket on too. Isn't that just fine?? I'll be below 200 yet. The funniest part of the whole thing is I don't feel any thinner. I'm wondering if I actually weighed 210 when I was home.

Darling, you're such a nice woman even though you cheat in Rook. Ha! Ha! You don't cheat when I play with you so I guess Sister must be a bad influence over you. Ha! Ha! But, don't worry, I love you just as much as ever even more if that's possible.

Honey Bunch, I have to laugh every time I read your letter in which you tell me about taking Sister down to Schlegel the other Sunday. Turning "down" at 5th and Walnut really was a "boner", wasn't it??? I just wonder what that "cop" was thinking of when you turned right. He must have been in a "daze". Did you go all the way down to 4th St. on Walnut?? Dearest, did you listen to your hubby and use the car for work this week?? If you didn't were you able to make the 5:30 bus?? I'm glad the other two people are nice.

[Wednesday] November 7th

Today I have some news that may interest you. We stood formation at 6:30 this AM and the First Sgt. read off the names of six men who have between 36 and 39 pts. These men are going to leave on Saturday, and they're going to

Camp Swift, Texas to join the 2nd Infantry Division which is training there. After Saturday, the only group who have not been told where they're going is the 40 to 50 pt. group. I'm hoping since I was declared essential after everyone leaves, I'll be sent to my reception station.

Darling when you call your gynecologist and he finds that there is nothing the matter with you, ask him if there is any way in which I can increase the number of cells or some way in which those cells of mine can make contact with your "egg". If he doesn't know that ask him if he thinks I should submit to some sort of examination whereby the condition of my fluids could be examined. We'll have to look into the matter.

My Honey Bunch, are you putting your medication in your eye regularly?? Do you think it's getting better?? I believe maybe your nerves caused that "flareup" of scar tissue because you were so upset during the spring of this year when I was in that "campaign". Did he test the sight of your eye?? I believe he is a good Doctor. He doesn't aim to get all the money from you he can.

Did my Sweetheart vote yesterday?? Darling, the "polls" are open until 8 PM. Even if you would have had to work until late you could have gotten up to vote before 8. Did your Daddy vote too?? The Democrats won a tremendous landslide in N.Y. City.

[Thursday] November 8th

Well, I've heard that it went over the radio that all 50 pt. men would be discharged during December. There is still nothing new on what I'll be doing or where I'll be going, once I leave here. I'm sorry, my Sweetheart if I seemed "blue" when they told me I couldn't get my Cpl. rating. It means absolutely nothing to me except the extra money and now I have this mail job with all the work and responsibility and no extra money for it.

That fellow Briggs was still here when I got back. He left the Saturday after I returned. He had to go to the hospital and spend a certain amount of time there before his discharge would come through. Then he caught the train home around 2 PM. He got home the following Monday and Thursday he started school at the University of Pennsylvania. He certainly got to work in a hurry, didn't he?? Boy is he a lucky fellow!!!

Darling, I'm really mad at you!! I told you to go see "Her Highness and the Bell Boy" last Thursday and you didn't go. Gosh, my Sweetheart just must go to see some movies. Now that's an order from the "boss". Do you understand that?? Ha! Ha!

[Friday] November 9th

Dearest, something came up this noon that I guess I'll have to tell you. My Ltd. told me that I should apply for a Dependency Discharge. Somehow, I got talking about my father's condition and he almost insisted I apply for such a Discharge. I told him that I didn't think it would go through. Well, he said there isn't any harm in trying and he will talk to my Captain about it too. Here is what is required. You must present at least three letters. They should come preferably from a Doctor, a Minister, and any other person who knows the existing conditions. The letter from the Doctors and Minister must be notarized. They should contain the condition of the individual and the need for which I'm required at home. He also asked if I could include you in my dependency plea. He said that would really clinch the matters. Ha! Ha! These letters I'll present to a board which reviews and acts on them. I was told that quite a few men put in for such a Discharge and only a few have been accepted, so I'm

331

not expecting too much. I'll write home to Mother and Daddy about this. The trouble is Mother is the only one at home that can attend to matters and it's hard for her to see the Doctors. I guess she can call them and ask them to write a letter explaining Daddy's condition and why I should be home. Personally, I'm not much for asking for something like that but I felt you would want me to and the Lt. practically insisted that I write home for the letters.

This morning the whole Medical Detachment stood formation and our First Sgt. said that there was a very strong rumor circulating; that men with 40-49 pts. would receive 45-day furloughs and then report back to their reception centers and await discharge. Boy, what I wouldn't give to have one of those citations come through to give me 41 pts.

Yes, Honey Bunch, I can be glad that I took that course in Spectroscopy. It will mean a lot to me if I got back to Carpenter Steel. I'm quite sure my job is waiting for me, although there probably won't be as good work as during the war. I'm afraid Carpenter Steel is going to be hit pretty hard.

Well, how did my Honey enjoy voting?? Did they have the voting machines installed already??? According to Mother's letter, Loose and Kunkle won the school director posts. Well Anna lost out, didn't she??

[Saturday] November 10th

This morning I received two letters but this time there wasn't any there from my Darling Wife. Gee, but I felt so "empty". Your letter of the 7th must have been delayed along the way. One was a short letter from a fellow medic who was transferred to a Camp in Kansas. I believe I forgot to tell you I had received a letter from Herb. He's stationed in Springfield, Mo. You see they send me their addresses and then write a short letter.

Gee, I was busy practically all day. There is so much mail to be forwarded with these men leaving and our First Sgt. gave me a pile of "file" cards this morning. They contained names of men who had been transferred from this unit while overseas and the personnel office wanted their home addresses. The mail was very heavy this morning and almost 50% of it was for men who had already left. I listened to part of the Army-Notre Dame football game about 12:30 to 2. Boy, Army slaughtered Notre Dame 48-0.

Say, did your folks have any rabbit or pheasant yet?? Mother writes that they had some up home already. I guess Frank shot a couple of rabbits. I don't believe my Honey likes rabbit or pheasant meat, does she?? Well, she doesn't know what she's missing. That meat is very good.

Dearest, would the folks at home like it if Daddy would take over the store?? I presume they would, wouldn't they?? No Homey Bunch, that's not selfish of you for not wanting to live in Leesport!! If you don't think you'll be happy there we naturally wouldn't live there. Maybe your father wouldn't want me to go in business with him. After all, I believe one man can run the business by himself. Of course, we'd fix things up and there would be lots of work connected to it. Yes, I think when we build, we should build with the whole family. If we leave up home, they'll be alone and it's just too much for Mother. We'll have to talk things over when I get home. Right now, the thing uppermost in my mind is to get home to stay. How about it?? Ha! Ha!

Dearest, are you annoyed with me to have mentioned the possibility of getting a Dependency Discharge?? Believe me, I wouldn't have if my Lt. hadn't insisted that I do. Now please don't get excited about it. If you can help Mother get the letters, I'm sure she'd appreciate it.

It was quite "nippy" again today. I guess the warm weather has left us for the year.

[Sunday] November 11th

It was today a week ago and just a few minutes earlier that I heard my Honey's voice, and gee, it makes me feel good just to think about that. If you felt as good about it as I did it was certainly worth every cent we paid. By the way, did they get the bill yet up home? I presume not but I'm certainly anxious to know how much it cost. I think it would be a very fine idea if you would pay for "half" the call. I'll pay you then myself.

Was my Darling in Sunday School and church this morning??? I'm sure she was. Were there any more discharged servicemen in Sunday School?? Say, is William still home on furlough?? I guess he'll soon be going back if he is. Now that the points have been dropped to 50, I guess he'll also be getting out. Well, one of these days they'll drop them to 36 and Snyder will get out. How about that?? Ha! Ha! Ha! Ha!

Gosh, the barracks I'm in is getting empty. There's hardly anyone around anymore. A fellow just came in and told me the men who are going to Camp Swift are getting a 15-day delay. Gee, I wonder if they'll send me to Swift too after everyone has gone.

How are you and that man at the beauty shop getting along?? I can't imagine a man working on women's hair day after day. I couldn't stand anything like that. At times when you think you'll have to stay late, you should absolutely use the Chevy.

Darling, are you sure you don't need that allotment check?? After all, you'll need money now to buy Christmas gifts. I wish I was home and could help my Darling with our

Christmas shopping. Well, at least I hope I'm home to help celebrate Christmas with her. That just about would be the happiest Christmas we ever spent, wouldn't it?? We're very lucky and we have such wonderful folks and friends. We do have much to be thankful for, don't we??

[Monday] November 12th

Are you celebrating a holiday at work?? I guess Armistice Day the stores and shops do not shut down, do they? Here at Camp, there is no training schedule being followed. It's another "Sunday" for everyone. Of course, I have my work just like any other day. That's one thing about being a mail clerk that isn't so nice. I'm still missing your Wednesday letter and the one you wrote Friday. Isn't that the funniest thing?? Some mail clerk must be loafing along the line somewhere. Ha! Ha! I'm sure it isn't the one at Camp Carson. Ha! Ha!

Darling, you are a bad girl!!! Why are you worrying about me??? If I would have known that what I wrote about those 36-39 pt. men going to Texas would worry you I never would have mentioned it. Dearest, I'm not in that group anyway. I'm not at all afraid of going overseas again, even if I do have to go to Camp Swift. This morning the clerk at the Regional Post Office said we would remain here until every man in the whole Regiment has gone. I think being essential will give me a break.

Thanks for sending me the results of Tuesday's election. I'm wondering how my Sweetness voted. Of course, strictly speaking, that is none of my business. Maybe she told me in Wednesday's letter which I'm still missing.

All three of Harold's boys were in the service!! I had a feeling they were. I knew Harold had some children but I didn't know how many. No, Ralph doesn't have any. Were they in the service very long??

What is Russell doing now?? Had he just gotten out of the Army when you spoke to him? Yes, that was quite a number of discharged men in Sunday School last week. That'll be a happy day for all of us when I can put on my civilian outfit again. What a day!!!

Say, did you receive any bonds yet? I think that the September bond should soon be coming through. I'm wondering sometimes if maybe they gave me the money instead of the bond because I certainly got more money than I should have last time. I even got more than I should if I'd get Corporal pay. Maybe my rating came through but since ratings are frozen, they didn't hand a written order down. That's been done before, I've been told.

[Tuesday] November 13th

Things are really happening fast here at Camp. At 9 AM the men below 40 pts. left for Camp Swift. Late this morning I moved to another barracks. The Medical Detachment is all in one barracks now and we don't even fill that one. The First Sgt. told us that the order came out that men with 40-49 pts. would be assigned to a "Special Troop" outfit of the 2nd Army which is stationed her in Camp Carson and from there would be assigned to various other outfits. Some 50 pt. men would still be here after they leave and myself. Either tomorrow or Thursday the Medical Detachment of the 85th Regiment will be no more. The men who are still here will be transferred to some Infantry Co. in the Regiment, probably Co. K. With no more Medical Detachment my job as mail clerk would be over, I'd think, but they told me I'd still retain my job. Yes, if I didn't have this mail clerk job, I'd be on my way to Texas right now.

This morning I went over to the Personnel Office and spoke to the officer in charge concerning a discharge. I told him the whole story and he said I had a very good case. He said that it all depended now on how impressive the letters were, on how well they explained the existing conditions, of how much I'm needed at home. I asked to go before the board personally because they read so many letters and really might not realize from the letters just how conditions are, but he said it's against Army regulations for a man to appear before the board. The point is now to get me the letters as quickly as possible so that I can present them to the board. He said, however, that having only 36 pts and less than two years of service might be a detrimental factor.

[Wednesday] November 14th

Well, Darling, I moved again. The Medical Detachment was dissolved and we were all transferred to one of three companies-Co. K, F, or B- I have been transferred to Co. K.

Sweetheart, in your letter of Friday, you mentioned buying those capsules that this woman claims makes one more fertile. Do they contain Vitamin E?? If so, I'd say they are O.K. because Vitamin E stimulates the reproductive organs. Gosh, I should have thought of that myself. You bet they are worth a try.

Darling, is Mother getting those "letters" together? Are you helping in any way? I only hope I'm not causing any of you too much work.

[Thursday] November 15th

Last night after I was finished writing my letters, I put some dirty clothes in the sink in the latrine and let them soak. Then I took a shower and shaved. You can't send anything to the laundry anymore, that's all closed. I sent a set of O.D.s to the Quarter Master Dry Cleaning located right here on the post. I got them back Tuesday and they did a pretty good job.

It cost me $.40 ($.25 for the pants and $.15 for the shirt). That certainly wasn't expensive, was it???

I attended to my mail chores, as usual, this morning. The men who were in the Medics are so afraid they won't get their mail as regularly and as quickly through the Co. they are assigned to, so they come and ask me to get all the mail as before and they'll come to me for it. I handed in all the reports and records of Registered, Insured, and C.O.D. mail to my Captain and he thanked me and congratulated me in the way I ran the mail "business". He checked all the records and couldn't find a single error.

As far as I know, no men were transferred from the Regiment today. I understand there was a shipment ready to leave for Ft. Dix, New Jersey but they couldn't arrange for any trains until Sunday. There isn't anyone left here with less than 40 pts., I'm the only one.

So, my Darling still is reading such "sexy" books?? I never thought my wife would read things like that. What would you think of your hubby if he read such things? I never got any further than detective books. Ha! Ha!

Yes, my Sweetheart, I got Grandma a birthday greeting when I was in town, at the Walgreen Drug Store. I'm satisfied with you buying her that nightgown, I'm sure it's very pretty. Did you have ice cream and cake when you went up home?

Darling, I'm going to "spank" you for worrying about what to buy me for Christmas. Honestly, I don't know that I need anything. I'm sure that whatever you get I'll enjoy it. You bet my Dear things are really going to "pop" when I get home. Don't you worry about that!! When I move to my next Camp, I'll have you send me some of those Vitamin E pills then I'll be all "set" when I get home. Ha! Ha!

That was cheap for that lot Daddy and Mother bought across the street. It's a real nice lot too.

[Friday] November 16th

Well, I received the letters from the Doctor, Minister and all the rest of the people. Sister had sent me one too. Gee, that was nice of your father to write one too. In all I had eight letters and believe me they were all very fine.

Quite a bit happened today so I think I'll start at the beginning. This morning I overheard the head mail clerk tell one of the unit clerks that he was taken off the essential list. He said that Regimental Headquarters complained that with so few men left in the Regiment there were too many mail clerks. He said he was told to recommend six mail clerks to be taken off the list. After he was finished talking to the fellow I asked if I was one of the six. He said no but since the Medical Detachment had broken up, he didn't know how long he could hold me essential.

Well, I realized that once I would be taken off the list I'd soon be shipped out and I wanted to have those "letters" turned in before. As soon as the Personnel Office opened, I went over and showed the letters to the officer. He said I certainly had a good case and then asked me how many points I had. Then he said that all men with less than 40 pts. were supposed to be shipped out immediately, essential or not. He then called up Divisional Headquarters and asked them not to put me on orders because I'm going to make an application for discharge. Then I had to write a letter myself and have it signed by my Commanding Officer. Tomorrow morning my "case" goes before the Divisional Reviewing Board. I've been told that it sometimes takes over a week before you hear one way or the other. Now please, please don't count on this going through because I think my chances are very slim. If I hadn't made an application today, I'm afraid I would not have been able to do it later.

I certainly do appreciate what you did, my Dear, toward getting the letters. I'm sorry that you missed the 1:30 bus simply because of Dr. Spamuth's letter not being ready, plus all the running around you did in going to the Red Cross. I'm sorry to have caused you so much work for nothing but you never know, there's always a chance.

[Saturday] November 17th

Gee whiz, by the end of next week I'm afraid practically the whole outfit will be gone. Right before noon today a lot of men received orders to be shipped out. My name was not among them so I'm sure I won't leave until my application is voted on and that will take at least a week. Those men that are leaving are being shipped to camps in the midwest around Missouri, Nebraska, and Minnesota.

This afternoon I was listening to some football games and Army beat Penn by a terrific score of 61-0. That Army team just can't be beaten.

Honey, did you take any of those Vitamin E capsules yet?? I'm very nervous to have both of us use them. I'm sure they won't do us any harm and I believe they could have a good effect. Don't you want to start taking them before I get home??

Dearest, I must laugh when you described those two people you are working with. So, they're both very religious?? How old is the man?? He really must be a little "cuckoo". Any man that gets manicures and especially permanent waves must be a little "touched". Ha! Ha! Does he speak French and German in the shop?? I'm so glad my Darling likes her work better than she did the other shop.

Sweetheart, I'm sure that you are feeling a lot better this Saturday than you did last week. I don't think I'll call up tomorrow because I have nothing new to tell you. If I'd have found out something as to my discharge or where I'll go to, I'd call home but I have no news.

I'm really glad that you don't feel "sore" anymore, my Dear, and I'm going to let you prove it the first time I see you. You aren't kidding when you say we're going to "town" when I get home. Things really will start popping when I get home, how about it?? Ha! Ha!

[Sunday] November 18th

Does my Sweetheart realize what day it is?? Probably not, but I thought about it yesterday and at midnight last night I started home from Camp Barkeley 52 weeks ago. I called up my Darling at work. Remember??? If we knew at the time what was to follow, I'm sure we wouldn't have felt so good, would we?? Well, all that is the past and the future looks much brighter, doesn't it??

At 10:00 I went to church services. The chaplain said that this service would probably be the last one we'd have since we'll all be gone by next Sunday. It was more or less a farewell sermon. He spoke of us being together as a unit in battle and at church for a long time. It was a rather impressive service. If I'm here yet next Sunday, I guess I'll have to look for another place to go to church.

Gee, I had lots of mail this noon that had to be forwarded. Men who left two weeks ago are still having mail come here. Your Friday letter was postmarked 12:30 PM and I got it at 11 AM Sunday. Gee, you complained in that very letter about your mail reaching me so irregularly and I get that letter in less than 48 hours. That letter made excellent time.

This morning and this afternoon up until I started your letter, I was reading the paper. This noon we had chicken again for dinner, mashed potatoes, corn, lettuce, cocoa, sliced peaches, and ice cream. It was very good and I ate too much again. Ha! Ha! But I won't eat any supper now. That'll make up for all I ate for dinner.

The first rumors that spread had all men below 40 pts would be sent to Camp Swift. Then a rumor also went out that the 2nd Infantry Division was going to relieve the 86th Division in the Philippine Islands. Soon another rumor came out that they were going overseas. Honestly, you absolutely can't believe anything you hear. 99% of all these rumors are false. I'm glad now that my Sweetheart is feeling better about everything. You need not fear that I'll go overseas.

By golly, there must be a way for me to get more "cells". If that's what's keeping things at a standstill, we'll have to do something about that.

Rev. Stoudt had church this morning, didn't he?? I'm sure my Sweetheart was there as well as in Sunday School. Was Potteiger in Sunday School?? Did you see Santilli too?? The boys are starting to come home pretty fast now. Well, that's mighty fine. We'll all be home before much longer.

[Monday] November 19th

I heard this morning that the Division is accepting no more applications for discharge. Some men had just received their letters from home and they refused to accept them but told the men to make applications at their next camp. The way things look I just got in "under the wire". Ha! Ha! Well, I'm another day closer to finding out what the results will be, and yet I'd be willing to bet that I'll be rejected. Oh well, at least I made an effort.

This morning about five truckloads of men left and later this afternoon I hear some more are leaving. Just before I started your letter, the rumor spread that all 50 pt. men would be sent to Fort Logan, Colorado this week to be discharged. I also understand that the majority of 40 to 50 pt. fellows will be sent to Camp Campbell, Kentucky to join the 5th Infantry Division. Gee, Kentucky wouldn't be too far from home, a lot closer than Colorado or Texas. Of course, I only have 36 pts. Ha! Ha! I'm wondering how soon I'll leave here once my application is rejected. Ha! Ha!

Did you have any more trouble with the Chevy not starting??? I can't see that the battery water should have been low already. Didn't I have the car greased and the oil changed when I was home? They (Stoudt) always check the water in the battery. I've never checked the battery since I've had the car. I surely hope you didn't have any more trouble. Darling, you mustn't be afraid of anything happening to the car when you're driving at night. That's all imagination!! No one will "hold you up". Ha! Ha! No, Sweetness, I don't think you're a baby at all. You're the Most Wonderful Wife in all the world and I love you so very, very much.

So, my wife would like to have five children!!! Okay, five it will be, you know you're the boss. Ha! Ha! I think we'd better start to get to work on "it" don't you?? As I said before things really will "pop" when I get home or I want to know the reason why. Your Mother's cousin is raising a big family, isn't she?? Heavens, that's 14 children; that fills a home doesn't it???

I guess my Darling doesn't have to work on Thursday, does she? I'll bet you'll have an excellent Thanksgiving dinner. I don't know what we'll have but I'm sure it'll be good.

[Tuesday] November 20th

Holy smokes, but the weather has made a change out here. Yesterday I told you it was so warm. Well, it's exactly the opposite today. It's frightfully cold. This morning when I got up it was very cloudy and as I was taking the outgoing mail down to the post office it started to snow. In no time everything was white. About 10:00 it stopped and seemed to get a bit warmer. Now it's cold and windy and it's snowing again. I guess I'm still a child but I really am fond of snow. Ha! Ha! You married a funny man, my Dear!!!

I'm writing here at the Service Club. It's so much nicer than in your barracks. They have a big room here with nothing but tables at which to write. It's very quiet and comfortable. Gosh, there are so few soldiers in it. I've heard that on Saturday, the Service Club will close because of all the men in the area left.

This morning at 5:45 a group left. That's pretty early to have to pack up and leave, isn't it??? There are still all sorts of rumors flying around as to when and where everyone is going.

Dearest, they never told me here that I needed a letter from either you or Mother. Nothing was mentioned either about having one from my employer. However, one of the questions asked on this one questionnaire I filled out was my civilian occupation. I put chemist. The Red Cross was entirely right about how they might contact them in case they wished to investigate further.

Darling, did Flush bite you very badly?? Gosh, I'm so glad to hear that she's "nicer" in the last few days. I don't know what in the world to do to train her differently. She's such a cute dog too. Has she bitten Mother or Daddy lately???

How is the paper situation?? I guess you still don't have an Eagle or Times, do you?? So, the company is paying all their employees their full salaries during this whole controversy!! Yes, it's only the subscribers themselves that get a "raw" deal. How is the truck strike coming along??

So, you like this paper. You can buy it at the PX but I got practically a full box from a fellow who went home on furlough. He re-enlisted for a year but first got a 60-day furlough. He said he didn't need the paper and gave it to me.

[Wednesday] November 21st

Another shipment of low point men left for Camp Swift today and I would have been on that list if I had not applied for a discharge. About 250 to 300 men from the Division are leaving tomorrow and Friday for Camp Logan, Colorado to receive a discharge. All of them are 50 pt. men. I understand all 40 pt. men will leave Saturday or Monday probably to Camp Campbell, Kentucky.

This noon I was getting to feel rather anxious as to what happened to my application for discharge so I walked over to the personnel office and that place is a "madhouse" today. They are getting all the records of these 50 pt. men together and packing them to send to Fort Logan. I did manage to get a word with Lt. Terry. He said he hadn't heard a thing about me, then another officer asked me my name, asked the clerk if anything came down from Division on Snyder and the clerk said no. This officer said he'd call up Divisional Headquarters and inquire but they're closed on Wednesday afternoon and will be tomorrow too so I won't find out anything before Friday. I know, however, it definitely has not been rejected yet or they would have sent word down. Gee, with everyone leaving I'll soon be the only fellow around. Ha! Ha! Ha!

Dearest, I'm sorry you sort of expected a call from me on Sunday and didn't get one but really, I had no news at all. I figured I'd save such calls until I hear some "big" news. I'm sure Herb won't have his wife come to him because he expects to be discharged at least by the 1st of the month. He never said how he liked Missouri.

It doesn't matter to me where you get the Chevy inspected. How does the radiator work now?? Have you added any water or "solution" yet?? Is the battery O.K.? Does the car start alright??

Dear, I just can't think of a Christmas list to give you. I have everything a person needs or wants. Gee but you know your husband isn't "fussy". Any little 5 or 10 cent article will be sufficient. Ha! Ha! Gee whiz, I have to start thinking about what to get my Sweetheart too. Christmas will be here before you know it.

[Thursday] November 22nd

How is my Honey Bunch spending her Thanksgiving Day?? Were you up home at all?? How many big meals did my Darling eat??? Ha! Ha! Last night before I fell asleep, I couldn't help but realize how much we had to be thankful for. We're so lucky for all the blessings of life. So much could have happened in the last year and didn't. This is our first peaceful Thanksgiving in four years.

I was wondering early this morning if we weren't going to have some kind of church service today and about 9:30 a fellow who bunks right across from me asked me if I'd go to church with him at 10:00. He said he heard there were services at that time in the chapel. We walked down to the chapel but it was locked and we couldn't find anything more about services so I didn't get to a Thanksgiving service.

Darling, I'm sure you had a very good meal today but honestly, for the Army, I had an excellent dinner. I'm sure it was the best meal I've ever had in the Army. We had turkey, mashed potatoes and gravy, plum pudding, bread filling, peas, salad, pumpkin custard, candy, and each fellow had a pk. of cigarettes at his seat. (I naturally gave mine away). I had three helpings of turkey and potatoes and two "milky way" bars. I was still eating when the K.P.s came around to clean off the tables. Ha! Ha! I've never sat down to a meal in the Army which looked quite like this. Everything was on the table and they filled the turkey platter over and over.

The Company K had invited the wives of any man in the Co. who had his wife in town to come to dinner. I thought that was a mighty fine gesture. One soldier had his wife and two small children there and gosh but those "tots" enjoyed themselves. Gee, it would have been wonderful if my Honey was with her hubby, but don't worry, I'm going to eat my Christmas dinner right beside my wife in Berks County. Mother wrote they had duck and oh my I wish I could have been there to help eat it.

Honey Bunch you must not get so angry because my mail doesn't reach me on time. After all, I did finally receive those two delayed letters and that's what counts and there for a while, your letters came through in less than 48 hours. Please don't worry, my Dear. I'll always know you're writing even if I fail to receive the letters on time.

Dearest, why should I mind if you go to the movies without me!! I've told you time after time to go to more movies. I know my Dearest behaves no matter who she's with or where she goes and now that you have such a nice person (Helen) to go with you I insist that you go more often. If only in some way Mother could go with you. She enjoys movies so much but she just can't get away.

I wish too I could go before the "board" and plead my case in person because those men receive so many letters to read and they all probably sound alike to them. But Lt. Terry said it was against regulations to do that. I'm hoping you and the rest of the folks aren't counting on me getting discharged because the chances are so very slim.

Haven't you received any bonds for us yet?? Depending on how much money I get at the end of this month I'm going to inquire into the matter. I want to know just where I stand.

I'm either not getting my bond allotment deduction or they're overpaying me or I'm receiving Cpl.'s pay. I feel that the former is what's happening.

I guess my letter got pretty long, didn't it?? Well, if my Honey enjoys my letters as much as I enjoy hers, I'm sure it won't be too long.

[Friday] November 23rd

I became so anxious again this noon, wondering whether or not the application was approved that I decided to go to the personnel office again at 1:00. Lt. Terry wasn't in. I asked about three clerks whether anything had come down or not and they said they still had no report on my case. This other officer who I talked to Wednesday was there so I asked him and he said he had no word either and that he wasn't going to call up Divisional Headquarters because he was reprimanded a few minutes before when he called, because of the number of calls the office was putting into Division. He said they'd notify me as soon as they heard one way or the other.

I noticed you had written that third page of your Friday letter up-side-down. I was going to kid you that you must have had something to drink and you were feeling a little "tipsy". I guess my Honey has taken to drink. Just kidding, my Sweetheart!!!

Why doesn't my wife like Camp Swift? Is it because of memories of where I went from there when I was there before?

[Saturday] November 24th

Boy, is it empty here!! I'd say there were close to 400 men who left the Division today and the place is beginning to look deserted. I honestly don't believe there are more than a dozen men left in our barracks anymore and I just heard that the whole 85th Regiment is going to be assembled into one Company on Monday. All still here then will move to Co. F so I presume my address will change to Co. F starting Monday. I presume most of the men who are still here have gone into town for the night.

I got another letter from Herb. He's written me two now and I haven't answered either of them. He begged me to write him. I guess I must write him a short letter sometime. He's anxious to know where all the fellows went to and how I'm getting along. He does not think he'll be discharged this year anymore and he feels pretty bad about it. He says they'll give him a 21-day furlough but he must spend either Christmas or New Year at his camp. He can only be home over one of the two holidays. Well, I know which one I'd select. Ha! Ha! I'm hoping I'll be able to spend both days in the arms of my Dearest Wife.

Dearest, I'm so glad to hear that you'd like to go to the Army-Navy football game. I'm sure you'd enjoy football much better if you several games and understood the object of the game. It's a very exciting game, but don't count your chickens before they're hatched. Ha! Ha! December 1st is only a week away and I'd say only a miracle would have me home next Saturday. Plus, I was always under the impression you had to put your order in for tickets months and months ahead of time.

I'm wondering whether we're going to have church services tomorrow morning. Gee, I certainly hope so but I'm very doubtful of it with so few men here they might have even transferred the chaplains already. I'm certainly going to try and find a church service somewhere on the Post. So, Rev. Stoudt has communion services on the 16th of Dec., that's two Sundays before Christmas. I certainly would like to be home for communion. The last communion I took was in July 1944 in my home church.

I listened to parts of the Philadelphia-Washington professional game. I guess my Honey gets disgusted at her husband and his sports doesn't she???

[Sunday] November 25th

Good afternoon my Sweetheart!!! It's almost 5 PM back home and I'm wondering what my wife is doing? She might be up home at this time and playing Rook. Since you have evening services today, you'll probably go up home late this afternoon and then go from there to church. Am I right??? Is my Honey getting tired of this stationary?? They have huge piles of it here at the Service Club so I took quite a bit of it. If it isn't good enough please tell me. My other paper is all gone and I never get to the PX to get any. The Service Club is about nine blocks from our barracks and it's a good twenty-minute walk but the exercise does a fellow good. There is absolutely no more training of any sort here at Camp. The men are just waiting to be transferred.

They asked me at the post office this morning whether I'm not on orders to leave yet. I said I hadn't heard a single thing. They said they were glad I was able to stay. I guess we'll all be out of here before too long.

This morning I went down to the chapel and we had services but there were very few people there. Counting the chaplain there were ten soldiers, four from our barracks alone. He had a very good sermon. The title was "Unconditional Surrender". It made a fellow stop and think and consider just whether he's living his life as God would have us live it. During my spare moments this morning, I read the Sunday paper.

Honey, Bunch, I'm certainly anxious for you to go to that movie at Lowes which has those good actors and actresses playing in the picture. Boy, that sounds like an excellent picture. Van Johnson and Walter Pidgeon are very good. I must warn My Dear again not to be so sure that I'll get a discharge. You're letting your imagination run away with you. It will be such a letdown then if it's rejected.

You seem to have expected another call from your hubby on Thanksgiving. I guess I spoiled you by calling a few weeks ago, didn't I?? I had no more news to relate. I haven't the slightest idea where or when I'm leaving here. You must just have patience. I know exactly what you mean by "suspense". After all, I'm right here and expect to hear at any minute what they've decided and now it's been about nine days and still no word. I believe in a day or two I'll know what the future holds for us.

So Henne was discharged!! Well, that's just fine. Had he gone back to his camp and then was discharged? I saw in the paper that by the middle of next month approximately 1/2 of the Army personnel will have been discharged. Many men took home or sent home many souvenirs of Italy and Germany. I had many opportunities to get things also but never thought they were worth having.

Did you say you'll call the Doctor about the 29th??? That's this week. You'll ask him won't you if there's any way I can increase my cells. If there's any medication I can take or treatments or even a change of jobs, believe me, I'll do it. Anything whereby it'll help us have children I'll gladly do. Dearest, would you like me to take those vitamin E pills right now??? As soon as I get to my next camp you send me some and we'll start taking them immediately. Maybe by the time we see each other then they will have "enriched" us. How about it?? Ha! Ha!

Don't you worry, my Dear, we'll go on long walks when I get home. We'll also go to see some Hockey games too. I sure hope to get home on a furlough before the Hockey season closes. We'll see plenty of football, basketball and baseball games. We're going to raise lots of children and be oh so happy together. I certainly would like to be in Philadelphia this afternoon to see that game between Philadelphia and Washington.

So, my Sweetness is considering buying a new winter coat and maybe even a fur coat at that!!! Well, that's perfectly alright. The only thing is I wouldn't let having me get a discharge influence you one or the other because I'm afraid if you do you won't get a coat. My Wife is being too sure of me getting out. I just can't believe I'd ever get a break like that.

[Monday] November 26th

My Dearest said she has had so many headaches lately. She never was bothered with such things. Do your eyes pain you?? Dearest, you absolutely must not let this "suspense" pray on your nerves. It isn't worth it. This morning I again went over to the Personnel Office. Nobody will be shipped out of this camp before Thursday and no orders will be issued. They admit that my application is taking quite a bit of time but there is nothing I can do but wait. I have some more news that I think will please you. I've been told by personnel that under all circumstances I'll be shipped to Camp Campbell, Kentucky if the application is rejected. They will not send me to Camp Swift. I think that's a pretty good break, I can easily get home on a 3-day pass from there and even if they won't give any furloughs over Christmas, I'd surely come home on a weekend and a 3-day pass combined. Well, that makes me feel pretty good, and here is something else. There is a rumor spreading that we might be shipped there "on our own" since there are so few men left and not enough to make up a troop train. If they do send us on our own, we'll be given seven or eight days to report to our camp. In other words, I'd come home for maybe three to five days on my way to Kentucky. I would travel on my own and the government reimburses you at 5 cents a mile from here to Kentucky. I have enough money to get home and spending those few days at home will not count against receiving a furlough later on. There is another rumor spreading the government aims to give all overseas veterans furlough over Christmas if at all possible. So, things look mighty encouraging today. Of course, I never become too enthused about anything I hear because things can change so quickly. Nothing I've said is absolutely definite except that I've got an inside tip that I'm going to Kentucky.

Darling, I don't know how often that "board" meets. I've been told however that everybody at Divisional Headquarters is very busy just now and that is probably why it is taking so long. Please, please don't think about me getting out so much. When I was over at the personnel office, they had just received the report on another fellow who had applied for such a Dependency Discharge and he was "rejected" so I'm afraid when mine is acted upon they'll vote the same way.

So, Grandma and Mother play against you when you play three-handed Rook!! Well, I must scold them for that. Did you and Sister give them any games yesterday???

Dearest, you really are the most wonderful wife any husband could possibly have. She didn't vote against the Amendment for sheriffs to succeed themselves because she thought maybe her hubby would someday be sheriff. Ha! Ha! Honey, that was mighty sweet of you, and believe me I appreciate that but I believe your hubby would be satisfied with one four-year term.

[Tuesday] November 27th

Well, things are still "humming" out here at Camp. Now instead of most men leaving on Thursday, we aren't going until Friday if I'm one of them. I understand that on Friday everyone who hasn't been shipped by that time will leave then so I surely won't have many more days to wait to find out how I made out.

So, my wife is thinking about going to a fortune teller to see whether or not her hubby is going to get out of the Army!! Ha! Ha! Did I have to laugh when I read that in your letter!!! Darling, you must not let this discharge prey on your mind. This is the way I feel. I maintain I won't get it and am not planning on it. Then if it does happen to be accepted it'll come as a surprise.

We moved from Co. K to Co. F yesterday. We had to pack all our things and carry them to our new barracks. The barracks I'm in are pretty full now. Before we moved, we had to clean our barracks thoroughly. Since I've come to Camp Carson after my 30-day furlough I've been in five different barracks. I really get around, don't I?? Ha! Ha!

How is our Christmas shopping coming along?? My Honey seems disgusted with shopping. Sister wrote that she too has had a difficult time finding gifts. Don't the stores have much to select from?? Well Dear, just don't worry about gifts. Remember it's not what you pay or how good the gift is but the spirit in which it's given.

Gosh, but I think that's a swell idea our parents have (and you as well) of putting a nickel a day aside for "tree accessories". Gosh, I hope and pray our parents will have a very happy Christmas. Are you going to have a big tree down home?

That was certainly nice of Mr. Bowman to take you along to Reading last Wednesday morning. I'm glad too that you finally went over to see Virginia. She certainly must have been anxious for you to come over. Is her husband still in Europe? Doesn't he have enough points to get out since he can add twelve to his total since the baby was born? I believe all 50 pt. men are supposed to be returned to this country by the end of the year. Is Clyde still in Europe and Francis?? Gosh, he has 70 points. He should be coming home soon.

I'll bet that dress material you got Mother is real pretty. Well, you have gotten quite a few Christmas presents after all. You know every year you think you'll never get it all done and before you know it, they're all bought.

So, William and I have been nominated and elected as Deacons again!! They didn't give us an opportunity to decline the nominations, did they?? Are they going to install us "in Absentia"?? Ha! Ha! They might have to wait quite a few months to install me in person.

Dearest, maybe the Chevy battery is getting weak. That battery has been in the car since April 1942. I got a new one after I had my license revoked. Remember?? I haven't bought one since. If you'd use it more often, she wouldn't run down as quickly.

Oh, but I love my Snookums so very, very much. She's the Dearest and Best Wife in all the world. We are so lucky to have such a great love for each other.   Love Luke

[This was the last posted letter in the tan cardboard suitcase. The Dependency Discharge must have been approved. Luke no doubt made his phone call to his Dearest Sweetheart and then jumped on the first train out of town. Christmas of 1945 had to have been a magical celebration not just for Luke & Ruth, but for all the Veterans and their families in the U.S and throughout the world.]

CPSIA information can be obtained
at www.ICGtesting.com
Printed in the USA
BVHW071032070521
606668BV00001B/45